HOW TO SMUGGLE CHILDREN AND OTHER

Confessions of a Country Doctor

DR. DAVID L. COGSWELL

◆ FriesenPress

One Printers Way
Altona, MB R0G 0B0
Canada

www.friesenpress.com

ISBN
978-1-03-914453-8 (Hardcover)
978-1-03-914452-1 (Paperback)
978-1-03-914454-5 (eBook)

1. Biography & Autobiography, Personal Memoirs

Distributed to the trade by The Ingram Book Company

Foreword

I was giving an anaesthetic for a difficult case while a local dentist operated.

He took a quick break, looked at me, and said, "This could only happen here in Nova Scotia."

"What do you mean?" I questioned, not comprehending.

"Well here I am, operating on my cousin!"

I stopped, looked at him and answered, "Doesn't seem strange to me . . . He's my cousin as well!"

This exchange made me realize that all professionals, including family physicians, who return to work in their small home communities are given the privilege, and the responsibility, to provide care for relatives. Inevitably some medical situations will be especially difficult. When almost all those in a small community are lifelong acquaintances—friends or relatives—there may easily be misunderstandings.

I represent the last of three generations of country doctors, all of whom have lived and worked in the same community in Nova Scotia. Our combined practices have spanned most of the twentieth century. It is interesting to think back about our practices—how they developed, how different we were, and yet how much alike.

Table of Contents

The Beginning

Home births were normal in the town of Berwick where I was born on October 20, 1936, and mine was no exception. My parents had built their house in Berwick the year before, and that is where I grew up, the first of six children. My father, Laverne Eidson Cogswell, and my maternal grandfather, Harold Edwin Killam, were both country doctors. I followed in their footsteps. Our three practices bridged most of the twentieth century. Although there was a hospital just a few blocks away, most babies were delivered at home due to the dearth of hospital resources, the cost, and because, at that time, home births were traditional. Prospective mothers were hospitalized only if complications occurred.

The Western Kings Memorial Hospital (WKMH) was opened June 3rd, 1922 as a practical World War 1 memorial. Berwick was the first town in the valley to have a community hospital, and beds were always in great demand.[1] At least one surgeon took the early morning train from Halifax, operated all day in this new facility, and then returned to Halifax on the evening train, leaving the post-operative care to local physicians. Prior to the construction of WKMH, any special examinations, procedures, or medical specialist consultations were available only by driving the three-hour trip to Halifax. Emergency surgeries were done on kitchen tables. In exceptional circumstances a few specific X-ray investigations might be permitted at the Nova Scotia Tuberculosis Sanatorium, twelve miles away in Kentville; everything else required the trip to Halifax. The hospital was upgraded with a new wing in 1951, which contained both laboratory and X-ray units, allowing investigations to be provided quickly and locally. We were fortunate to obtain a technician trained to do both X-ray and lab procedures when the new wing was opened. My father learned to take and develop his own X-rays and was also able to do certain lab tests, if the technician was unavailable.

Despite our Nova Scotian seafaring heritage, many people in the Annapolis Valley had never travelled even the distance to Halifax from where they had been born. My father had patients in his practice, many of whom were too fearful to take the trip to Halifax, even if they could have afforded it. Once in the city, they had no knowledge of how to find their way to the doctors' offices. In many of these cases, my father would make their appointments, take them in his own car to the Halifax consultant, and return them to their homes. In this manner, both my father and my physician grandfather carried on their practices. I followed naturally in their footsteps, absorbing their professional values, influenced by their actions and their stories.

After entering medical school, I was surprised to discover how little some parts of the curriculum had changed. One day my father unexpectedly appeared behind me. I was in the pathology lab, intently studying tissue through my microscope. When I asked how he had found me, he said,

"That's easy: the pathology lab was always on Thursday afternoons."

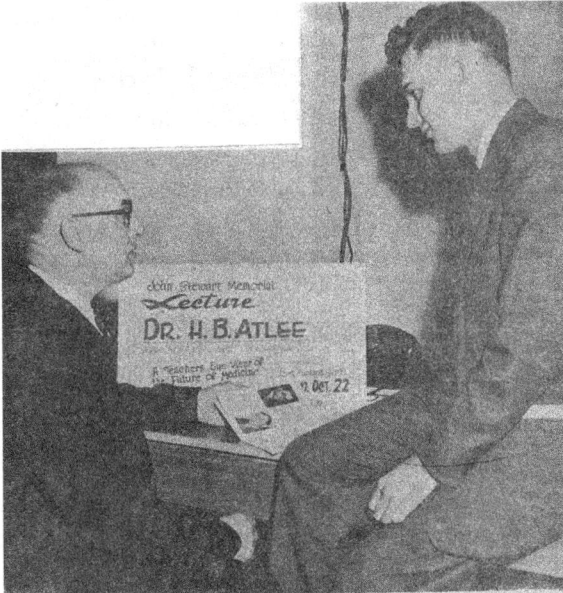

MEDICAL FAMILY — Dr. Laverne Cogswell, veteran practitioner of Berwick, and his 22-year-old son David, a fourth-year medical student at Dalhousie University, were two of the more than 100 medical people attending the opening of the 32nd refresher course at Victoria General Hospital Monday. The father and son combination, bolstered by another son, Eric, 20, in his second year of medicine, forms an unusual family in the field of medicine. The father, class of 1932 at Dalhousie University, has been practising in the Town of Berwick for 26 years. Dr. Cogswell's daughter, Elizabeth, 18, also is a student of Dalhousie University, majoring in biology. (Photo by Martin)

Dr. Laverne and Dr. David together
The Chronicle Herald, Halifax, N.S., October 25, 1958

My grandfather worked in WKMH from its inception, my father all his working life; and I worked there as well, until its closure in March 1996. Government funded medical care (MSI)[2] began on the 1st of April 1969, six years after I'd opened my practice. Prior to that, the costs of hospital care were a private responsibility. A few patients were fortunate and had medical insurance which paid both hospital and medical expenses. My grandfather was contemptuous of the forms requested by the insurance companies of the few patients of his who were insured. He preferred to relinquish his payment than "waste his time" filling out the forms. This forced my grandmother, who needed household money, to fill them out for him to sign. He

3

was mostly paid "in kind"; as a result, there was no money for his children's university education. My mother obtained scholarships to be able to attend both Dalhousie for her Bachelor of Arts degree and the University of Toronto for her Master of Arts degree[3]. Her name was on the front page of the provincial newspaper, revealing to all that her marks were some of the highest of the provincial high school examinations. My mother seemed to know everything. I was surprised as I grew up, that not every mother knew everything.

My mother and Margaret, her sister, were always together. Strangers often thought them twins. Margaret waited a year to start school so they could be in the same class. It was almost inevitable that they would be married in a double wedding, and this occurred on September 12th, 1935, when Kathleen Killam, my mother, married Laverne Cogswell, and Margaret married Carl Atwood.

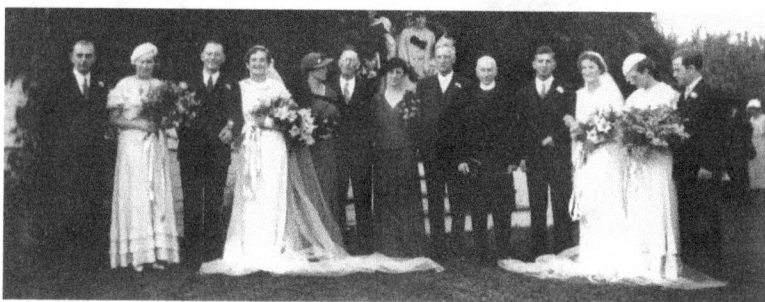

The double wedding of Harold and Ora Killam's daughters Kathleen (my mother) and Margaret was held at the family home in Woodville. Left to right: Gerald Nichols (first cousin to Laverne); Nan Chipman (later Robinson); Laverne E. Cogswell; Kathleen Killam; Margaret (Chute) Cogswell (Laverne's stepmother); Eidson Cogswell (father to Laverne); Ora Louise (Webster) Killam; Dr. Harold Edwin Killam; minister, Dr. F. R. Prince; Carl Atwood; Margaret Atwood; youngest sister Joyce Killam (later Barkhouse); Frank Lacey (Carl Atwood's best man)

My dad only had a couple of months to build a house for his bride, which would include his office. Conveniently, this was an opportune time to build, as the effects of the Great Depression still lingered, and he had been able to walk "uptown" and find excellent carpenters who were pleased to work for a dollar a day.

When visiting one Friday evening, he asked my mother how large a home she wanted, as he had carpenters coming the following Monday to begin constructing the cement basement. Mother often complained she was only given another week to design the remainder of their new home. The best building lot my father had been able to find on Commercial Street in Berwick was so marshy and wet he decided to pour the floor of the basement on top of the ground. The walls of the new basement protruded up exposed to the air, until wagon loads of topsoil built the lawn up to the proper street level. He expected to have a dry basement but was disappointed. The basement flooded in wet weather; even the unpaved street in front of the house became so deep with mud my uncle's car became stuck there at least once. When a new home was being planned for the lot next door, my father told the prospective owner about the wet land and suggested he not dig a basement. Years later he gave the same advice when another house across the street was being built. Both owners dug basements despite his warnings, and soon we saw water coming from their sump pumps. Following the installation of these sump pumps, our basement water problem improved immensely.

The Cogswells came to Nova Scotia as New England Planters. My branch settled on a farm in Morristown, five kilometres from Berwick on the South Mountain. Abner, my great grandfather, bought the property in 1863 and named it Maple Shade Fruit Farm. It was adjacent to his father, Oliver Hezekiah Cogswell's farm where Abner himself had been raised. They did mixed farming, apples being the largest crop. The two-hundred-acre farm had about fifty acres in cultivation and two houses, the "old house" and the "new house." The barn was the largest in Morristown. There was also a separate workshop-garage. The north side of the basement of the barn was designed to remain frost-free until after Christmas, allowing apples to be stored safely there for personal use and sale into the New Year. On many other farms, the stored fruit had long been destroyed. The land was fertile but very rocky. These rocks were cleared by hand using oxen pulling sledges. My grandfather, Eidson, used dynamite to blast rocks too large to be moved by the oxen. My university and school vacations were partly spent "picking rocks" in the manner of my ancestors.

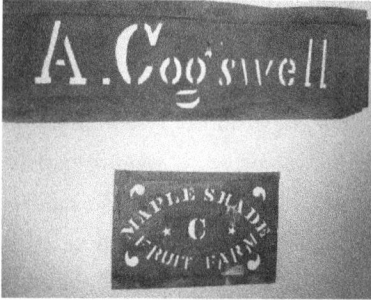

Abner's Apple Barrel Stencil
Cogswell Photo

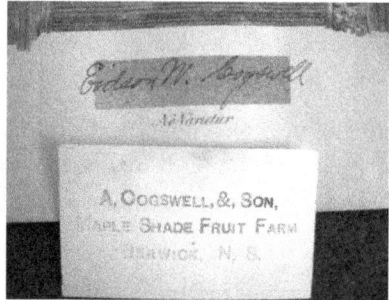

Abner Cogswell Stationary & Eidson's Signature
Cogswell Photo

My great-grandfather Abner Cogswell's stencil identified crates and barrels from the Morristown farm. His son, Eidson's signature is on the envelope. Morristown is a hamlet several kilometres south of Berwick, Kings County.

Eidson Witter Cogswell, my grandfather, decided that farming was a poor way to make a living. To augment his farming income, he became a 'shipper'. He sold dynamite to farmers who needed it to clear rocks from their fields. He bought their surplus produce, added his own and took his load to Halifax and other areas on a wagon pulled by oxen. He carried a revolver for self-protection when he returned home with a large amount of money. I remember him living in Berwick managing his farm and shipping from a home office, which contained a large safe for cash and records and the desk I now use. The day-to-day work on the farm was handled by a hired-man and his wife.

I remember running into my Grandfather Eidson on the sidewalk the first year I attended school. He was a slight, smallish man in a suit, vest and felt hat. I exclaimed, "Hi, Grandpa!"

He looked at me, tipped his hat in the same manner he tipped it to all those he met on the street, and greeted me with, "Good day, young sir."

Eidson encouraged my father, Laverne, an only child, to leave the farm and pursue a university education.

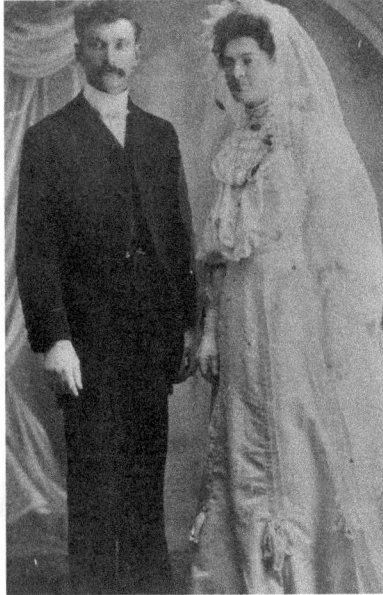

Eidson Witter Cogswell (1875-1948) and Naomi Elizabeth Nichols (1881-1927)
Wedding Photo, December 16, 1903

My father's mother, Naomi Nichols, died of "Graves' Disease" (hyperthyroidism) while Laverne was in university. She was a schoolteacher who loved gardening and was adored by all who knew her. She supported my father and urged him to continue his studies despite his dyslexia. Although she died before I was born, my father kept some of her last letters he received while at Acadia University. These letters reveal her support for his studies, her warm personality, and life as it was in those years. One, sent to him when he was attending Dalhousie medical school in Halifax, asked him to discontinue sending his laundry home on the train for her to wash, because the four-mile trip from Morristown to the train station was so muddy the wagon became mired in the mud.

Eidson's second marriage was to Margaret Chute, the only Cogswell grandmother I ever knew. She had been a milliner, making hats for the ladies in the town of Berwick where the couple now lived.

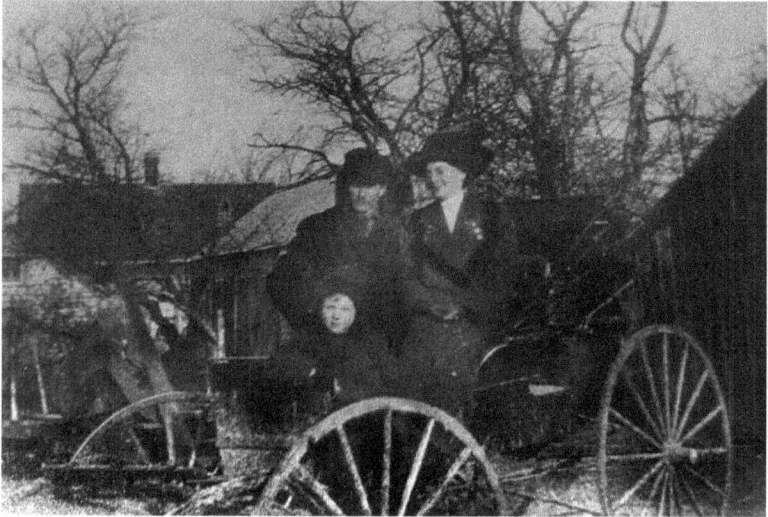

Eidson Cogswell and his wife, Naomi, with my father, Laverne, age three

Traditionally my family, and other relatives, had Christmas dinner with Grandmother and Grandfather Killam. It was a lively affair. Far quieter was our New Year's Day dinner celebrated with Grandma and Grampa Cogswell, as the only guests were our family of eight. One Killam Christmas was memorable because Grandmother dropped the turkey as she approached the dining room. Unphased, she simply picked it up returned to the kitchen and emerged with a turkey on a platter. 'It's a good thing I cooked two,' she said, not skipping a beat.

School Days

My five siblings and I reveled in the freedom and safety of the time. Our parents allowed us to wander all over town with other children in the area, who had the same privileges. All the adults knew each of us. Instinctively we realized we were secure, someone would send us home if we wandered too far afield, or if we fell and were injured our parents would be called. We lived close to the school and were required to return home for the noon meal, but many of our classmates carried lunches. We missed being part of the noontime camaraderie. Suppertime was announced to us, as well as all the neighbours, by Mother ringing a school hand bell that we children called the Cow Bell. Some of the neighbours complained of the noise, but its effective, loud call rapidly brought all six of us home, tired and hungry.

The September I was four, all my friends were excitedly preparing for school. There was no excitement in our home as I, the eldest, would not be of school age for another twelve school days. Although I had been told I was underage and would not be allowed to begin school that year, I did not really understand. Automatically, when my friends started school, I went as well.

The teacher called my mother and told her I was in the classroom. They were close friends, and both were certain I would quickly lose interest, so they decided to let me stay. I was given a desk for the day. However, I continued attending daily.

At the end of the year the class was told they had graduated and would be attending Grade 1 the next year. All except me. Since I had been there with my playmates unofficially, my schooling would only now officially, begin. Crying, I asked what I had done wrong; why was I being punished? The teacher decided to ignore my age and the rules and grade me with the rest of the class.

Our house, the "Doctor's House," was in the center of town, only two doors away from the movie theatre which provided entertainment from the outside world. Most of the films shown were Westerns. I vividly remember the owner smoking his nice-smelling cigars. On movie nights he sold tickets from a small, enclosed room through a window with a tiny opening. He'd then close the ticket office and become the usher, taking the tickets he had just sold. The moviegoers were finally allowed to enter the theatre and find their seats. He watched each individual carefully as they passed him. If their mouths were full, and especially if he found them chewing, they were required to leave their partly used chewing tobacco in the polished brass spittoon on the floor next to him. This may not have helped curb the spread of tuberculosis but it certainly made cleaning the theatre easier.

At that time, Western movies featuring "Indians" were hugely popular. This term seemed quite acceptable then, as we were unaware of its derogatory connotations. Our mother even made costumes, flaunting fringes along the sleeves of the arms and legs, complete with feather headdresses, for my brother Eric and me to wear in the annual children's Labour Day parade. We roamed the town in our costumes playing hide-and-seek.

Despite my love of movies, I attended them only as a special treat. I was saving my money to buy a bicycle. My mother was adamant I not own a bike. She had been hurt as a child, falling off of one, and was determined not to allow me the same fate. After some difficult and prolonged negotiations, she finally agreed to let me have a bike, but only if I earned the money to buy it myself. Later she admitted she thought her offer safe, since she did not think my small allowance would allow me to save enough for the transaction. I, however, being just as determined as my mother, managed to find a cheap second-hand bike needing a complete rebuild, which I carried home in pieces. I then found myself looking for parts and information in the only bicycle shop in town. Once Mr. Margerson, the owner, understood my predicament, he kindly gave me some used parts for free, and new pieces at very low prices. To show me how these new parts could be combined with what I already owned, he dismantled and reassembled similar parts in his workshop. After his demonstration, if I was still unable to do the assembly myself, he would do it for me. How fortunate was I, years later, to have the opportunity to return his kindness as his physician.

Now that we were energetic boys on bikes, my friends and I had the mobility to explore local businesses and to watch the activities inside. We learned how to sneak by the owners and visit certain special employees, who would covertly slip us treats. One of our favourite stops was a commercial bakery, a business only a block away from our house, owned by our next-door neighbour. My friend Billy and I were always hungry after school and automatically headed there. We knew from experience not to attempt to enter through the front entrance, where we might be caught by the owner who did not want the inspector to find us in the cooking area. Instead, we snuck in through the back, likely not fooling anyone. Our first stop was the man who made small cakes and pies. Anticipating our visit, he kept imperfect or damaged pastries for us. If none had been broken, he would slip us intact goodies, with the strong admonition not to let the boss see. Somehow these always tasted best, but we must have been seen, for one day he told us he had been instructed by the owner to give us only broken pies. "There are no broken ones today boys . . . oops! How clumsy of me—I just broke these two!"

In the fall we often indulged in another treat. The food processing plant was making fresh apple cider, and after the pies we were thirsty, so off we went to the far east end of town and found our way into the factory. I now realize we were very carefully watched while there, to prevent us from being injured by the moving belts and machinery. It was fascinating to smell and observe the apple mash as it was poured and wrapped in large cotton sheets in many layers. Hydraulic pressure then squeezed the juice through the cotton, forcing it to run out in rivulets. Until we were a bit older, the workers held the juice cans from which we drank, to prevent any cuts from the sharp edges of the cans or contamination of the juice. The best-tasting juice was the first pressed.

Not surprisingly, there were many orchards to provide apples for the pies and cider. The center of the block of houses across the street from us was filled with large mature apple trees. The largest of these trees was just behind my friend Billy's house. He and his older brother proudly constructed a treehouse high on the top of the tree, using ropes to pull the boards up and to secure them. My brother and I helped. This became the "boys' clubhouse." With my vertigo and difficulty with heights, I only managed to get up there driven by a lot of peer pressure, fear, and help. My younger brother got up much easier than I did. My sister, Elizabeth, three years younger, insisted she should be allowed up as well. "It's too dangerous," we four boys argued.

Mother, a strong feminist, insisted we had no right to restrict Elizabeth just because she was a girl. Mother was adamant: "Girls can do anything boys can do and should be allowed to."

Despite all our protests, we were compelled to relent. Horrified, we watched her perilous climb, but she made it.

After the leaves had fallen, the clubhouse became more visible. The flimsy structure constructed of boards tied to branches and a few nails was now easily seen from my mother's kitchen window, high above the neighbour's two-story house. Even the local dry goods store owner on the next street commented on the "crashed space-ship" visible from her store window. My mother said she regretted her decision to pressure us to allow Elizabeth to access the clubhouse now that she could see the danger, especially where we had to swing through the branches to get into it.

—

Chess, Hunting & Sailing

When I was about twelve years old, my grandfather Killam became a cardiac invalid and spent most of his day in bed. He needed assistance even to get into a chair. He was able to be up most afternoons for an hour or two, and again some evenings. Ora, my grandmother, would not leave unless he had a companion capable of providing his routine care and who was also able to look after him in an emergency. She planned most of her shopping and social visits for the afternoons when grandfather and his close friend, Mr. Mahar, were enjoying their twice-weekly chess tournaments.

To have some one-to-one contact with my grandfather, I decided to learn to play chess. This would allow me to be useful as a sitter and give us time to get to know one another as we concentrated on each other's moves. I learned chess basics from instruction books, studied them carefully, and then looked for someone with whom I could practice. I knocked on the door of a middle-aged woman who lived nearby and whose husband had a business on the home property. Apparently, she loved to play chess, and she agreed to teach me. For several months we both enjoyed our regular after-school chess matches. Then abruptly she announced, "This will have to be our last game as the neighbours are talking." It took me quite a few years to figure out why the neighbours were talking, and how their gossip could interfere with our chess matches.

I was now ready to challenge my grandfather. I made my offer for a combined chess match and babysitter visit, which received a lukewarm reception from everyone, my grandfather included. I persisted and finally, as an experiment, an afternoon was arranged. When I arrived he was still in bed. He made his moves rapidly, in a very casual manner. Much to his surprise, I won easily. "I want a rematch!" he declared. "Help me sit up! Get some pillows behind my back!"

Our relationship changed. From that day I was accepted as an adult. "Come over for a game," was the first thing I heard when we had our family visits. After entering university, I found neither the opportunity nor the time for chess, but I continued to consider myself a good player.

During my obstetrical internship at the Aberdeen Hospital in New Glasgow, very busy times alternated with quiet periods. I used the opportunity provided by the down time to be in the OR, learning from the anaesthesiologists and surgeons. I was accosted in the corridor one quiet evening, by the janitor who asked with a middle European accent, if I played chess. Pleased to hear I did, he invited me to play a game with him that evening. When I arrived in his basement office/workshop, he and a friend were already there, with chairs, table, and chessmen all in place. Apparently, it was their regular chess evening. I was given the place of honour, and in two or three moves lost in the first "fools checkmate" I had ever seen. I realized the janitor and his friend had carefully set me up. Did this happen to all the interns? I knew that even if I had continued with my after-school chess lessons, either of the two men could have easily and quickly checkmated me.

In junior high, I had briefly dated a girl in the class ahead of me. She and her older sister had tried to teach me how to dance, and her mother often baked cookies. I enjoyed my time there, but her father quickly put an end to my visits. I was not suitable, as I was Protestant, and they were strongly Catholic. This was my first episode of religious discrimination.

Later, one of this former girlfriend's children became my patient. During an office visit, I bragged to her I had just become a proud grandfather for the second time, and I asked how many grandchildren her mother had. She stared at me for so long I thought maybe I should not have asked this personal question during an office consultation. Finally, she said, "Twenty–one"; she had needed time to count. Her mother now has fifty or more descendants.

Even though the religious difference meant the possibility of a deep relationship was over, her older brother remained a friend and a sort of role model for me. He used his .22 rifle to hunt rabbits found mostly within the town limits. When he could afford a better weapon, he gave his old one to his sister, the one I had been visiting. She now owned a rifle, as did several of my out-of-town classmates. They all hunted rabbits which I was told was a delicacy. I had never tried it but decided to become a hunter and find out. My parents immediately made it clear I would not own a gun. To arm myself, I used long strips of bicycle inner tube rubber to make a slingshot, and, with the use of steel ball bearings, had a lethal weapon. Hunt as much as I could, I could not find any rabbits to shoot so I decided to use snares and organized a trap line which I attended daily. Finally, I caught a rabbit and proudly took it home. I had mixed feelings. It seemed mean to kill a rabbit and cruel to kill it in a snare, but I was bringing home the bacon.

My mother was appalled. "You want me to skin, clean, and cook that thing? You do it!"

I did not want to do it either and had quite a time giving it away. I never did develop a taste for rabbit.

Despite my loss of enthusiasm for rabbit hunting, I was still keen to have a dangerous toy. After all, many of my friends had the pleasure of owning their own firearms. I decided to build myself a crossbow from the plans I found in a *Mechanics Illustrated* magazine. I was certain I had the necessary skills, as I had been attending Camp Meeting's "Children School."

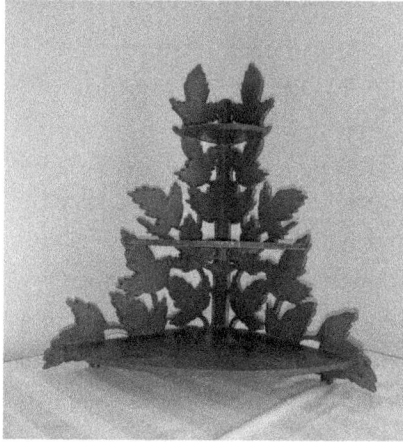

Knickknack Shelf made by me
Cogswell Photo

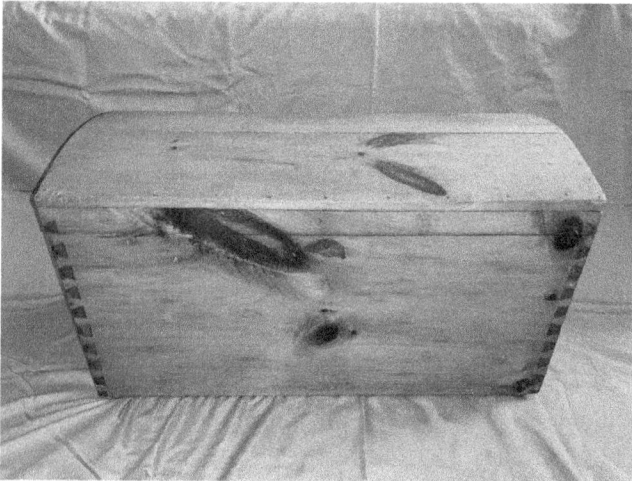

Sea Chest made by me
Cogswell Photo

"Camp Meeting" had been an integral part of summer in our town, for all age groups, since the first service on July 5th, 1872. Edward Foster, who had attended a summer religious evangelical camp while on a trip in the USA, decided a similar camp was needed in Berwick. With a core group of seven Berwick leaders, an area of the town that had never been logged of its hemlock trees was set aside for a church camp. "Camp Meeting" offered outdoor services and activities in an area conducive to meditation and worship. Cabins now replace the original tents, but active services continue to this day. Children are kept entertained, busy and quiet, doing crafts while the adults socialize and attend religious services during the ten-day summer camp. Here, as a child, I was taught to use a coping saw. My first project was a doorknocker in the form of a woodpecker, for my grandfather Killam. That winter, using my coping saw, I made a complex maple leaf ornamental corner shelf for my mother for Christmas. I also fabricated a lamp for my grandfather that now sits on my desk. The original lampshade is long gone, replaced by one made by my wife, Heide. I also made a sea chest with hand tools.

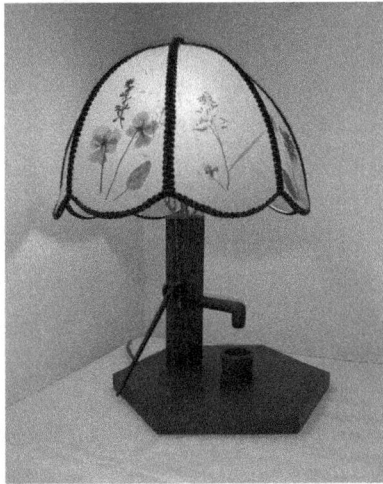

Water Pump Lamp made by me
Cogswell Photo

Now I needed to construct a crossbow. Little did the church camp leaders realize that the skills they had taught me would be used to make a lethal weapon.

My crossbow began to evolve: the stock was made from a beautiful piece of maple, the bow from the spring-leaf of an Austin car, and I bought solid bronze to make the fittings. The powerful bow broke these bronze attachments, and I had to substitute steel. The initial string was war surplus aeroplane cable, as the recommended bowstring cable could not withstand the tension. Later I was able to make a proper multi-stranded linen one. All this was done with hand tools. My uncle Fred Killam (brother to my mother who feared me riding a bicycle!) became interested and, despite my mother's protests, used his metal lathe to make the trigger mechanism. The "calking jack" I made of sturdy oak. Crossbow completed, I taught myself how to use it. A copy of *Time Magazine* became my target, but it needed to be backed up by a piece of three-quarter-inch plywood board, which prevented the bolt from going through the target into the wooden garage door. After a little practice and experimentation, I was able to hit my target. With more practice, and steadying my back against our neighbour's house, I managed to shoot across his lawn, the sidewalk, the street, up our driveway (missing our car), and only rarely missed my ten-by-twelve-inch target. When I did miss, I was sure to get a reprimand from my unhappy father. He always knew when I had missed, perhaps because my bolts would split the wooden boards of the garage door. Hazards, such as my five younger siblings, the patients entering and leaving my father's home office, our car in the driveway, or even the street traffic, never worried me. But I never did use the crossbow to hunt rabbits.

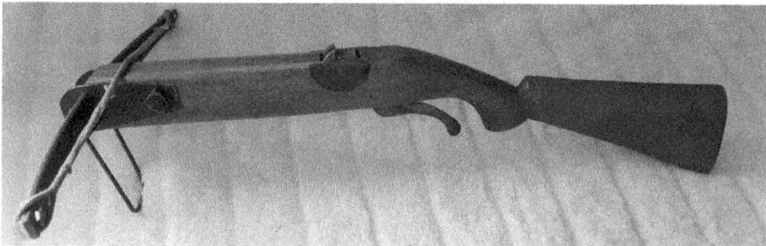

Crossbow made by me
Cogswell Photo

Emboldened by the success of my crossbow, I decided I needed a boat. Every summer we vacationed at Harbourville on the Bay of Fundy. There, I met Fred Merritt, who had an interesting collection of First Nations artefacts, including two antique birch bark canoes from Ontario, still in pristine condition. With a great deal of begging from me, and concern on his part, he finally allowed me the pleasure of paddling the smaller one-man canoe—but only in the harbour. The beautifully crafted canoe was watertight and floated high in the water. The birch bark shell was sewn to the frame with flexible tree roots but, as the frame was slightly curved, I needed to adjust my paddling to keep it going in a straight line. It was a privilege and an experience I have never forgotten.

When Fred took his turn with the canoe, his expert paddling was fascinating to watch. I was later just as amazed as he constructed a small sailing yacht. As this yacht seemed to magically appear it fuelled my wish to be on the water, but I did not have access to a boat. To be on the water I would have to construct my own watercraft. I found plans for a ten-foot sailing dingy in *The Young Craftsman* (1942), a book I had received for Christmas. Fred and I discussed the plans, of which he approved. He even suggested I could substitute larch (locally known as "hackmatack") boards my father had on the family farm, for the prohibitively expensive marine plywood required in the original plans. This free lumber would make building the boat financially possible for me. I could join the boards with shiplap construction, fabric, and marine glue. To save money I used galvanized-steel marine nails and tacks instead of copper screws. To avoid damage from electrolysis, I had to use one or the other, but not both. Saying he hated to see them wasted, my father reluctantly agreed to give me the boards.

I desperately needed money to buy materials for this boat-to-be and my other projects. I was lucky enough to get a Saturday job as a "striker" with Johnny, a bread truck driver-salesman. My job was to carry the Berwick Bakery products into the stores and put them on the shelves while Johnny negotiated with the store managers. On our way home we would stop the truck at a canoe manufacturing shop where I bought glue and nails. Noon lunch was a pint of milk each.

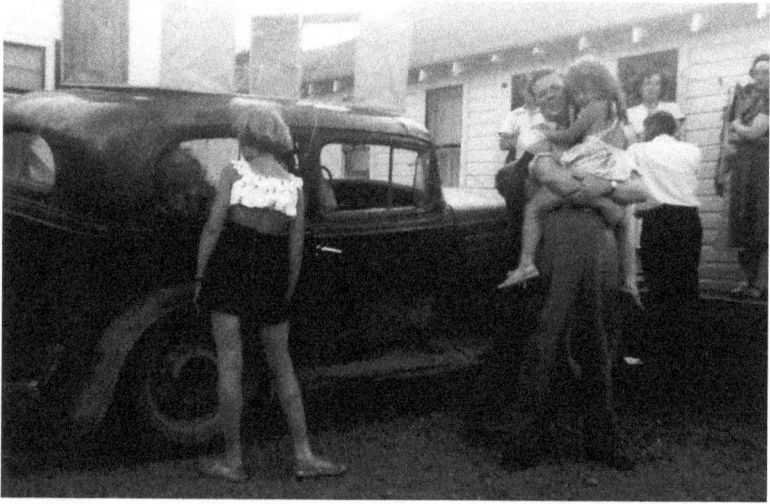

Box Kite on top of Fred Killam's car. Mary Graham (Cogswell) on left, Milton Barkhouse (Joyce's husband) holding Suzanne Cogswell, sisters Kathleen & Joyce watching from deck and their brother, Fred Killam with his back to us.

I set aside an area of the basement for my construction site. When finished, my boat would need to be taken outside or else become a permanent basement knickknack. I carefully measured the size of the opening of the platform at the top of the basement stairs, where a ninety-degree turn led into the garage and outside. The platform, level with the top of the basement stairs, also provided a base for other stairs, which led up into the house. If the partially-completed boat was tipped and turned carefully, I was certain there would be enough clearance to get it up the basement stairs, around the turn, into the garage, and outside. As the boat took shape, my parents and others who visited were not so sure. I confess I was worried as well and felt very lucky when, with only a few inches to spare, we carried my new boat outside, and I saw it in the sunshine.

To build my sail from rolls of factory cotton, I needed a sail loft. The largest room in the house was the living room, a perfect fit. My siblings and I had frequently conscripted this open living area for our large projects; the latest had been to manufacture kites.

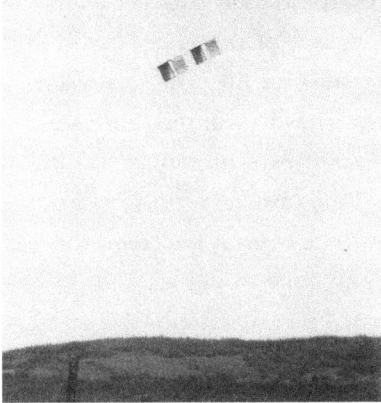

Box Kite

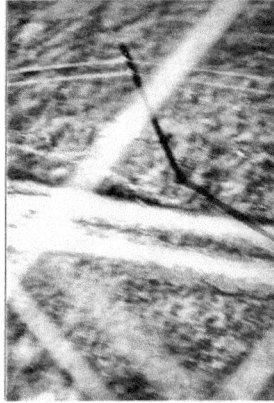

Picture of Telephone Pole from Box Kite

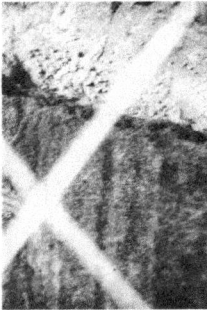

Picture of Harbourville Bluff from Box Kite

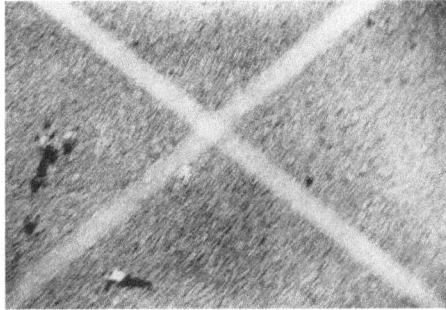

Picture of People from Box Kite

When my uncle Fred saw us building our kites, and our flying endeavours, he decided he and his children should join us. The excellent huge box kite he constructed far outdid our tiny ones. We realized it was large enough to carry my Kodak Brownie box camera and decided to try aerial photography, an unusual idea in those pre-drone days. Uncle Fred would contribute the kite, I the camera. The Sunday he arrived at the Killam family cottage in Harbourville for our first day of flight trials, he made quite an impression. The car was full of his children, with the kite securely strapped to the roof.

We decided to take aerial pictures of the Harbourville cottage. Because of our concerns for the safety of the camera, it was secured and balanced in the centre of the kite. To trip the shutter an aluminum tube was driven over the mooring string up to the kite, by a cardboard sail. When it reached the camera, a small parachute was unhooked; this, in turn, tripped the shutter and took the picture. Once the tube was on its way only luck would keep the kite in the desired position for the anticipated picture. There were gusty winds above the Killam cottage, and this made it difficult to maintain a proper position for the photographs. To take the next picture, the kite had to be brought back down, the film wound and reloaded, and the shutter release tube returned to the correct position. We waited four long days for the film processing to be completed, only to discover that the pictures had come out, but we had missed the cottage.

I now needed the space the living room provided for a sail-loft. I moved the furniture to its time-honoured, kite-construction, out-of-the-way locations. This gave me just enough space on the floor to glue the grocery store wrapping paper together, on which I outlined a full-sized sail pattern. Here I would assemble the sail. To sew together the many pieces of factory cotton, I asked my busy mother to teach me how to use her sewing machine. Looking forward to quickly finishing my sail, I began by breaking several of my mother's best needles, leaving her fearful the same thing would happen to her sewing machine. The living room had been in chaos for days with no end in sight, and my mother was soon to host her weekly bridge club. She surprised me by offering to speed up the construction by doing the sewing for me, and the sail was quickly completed.

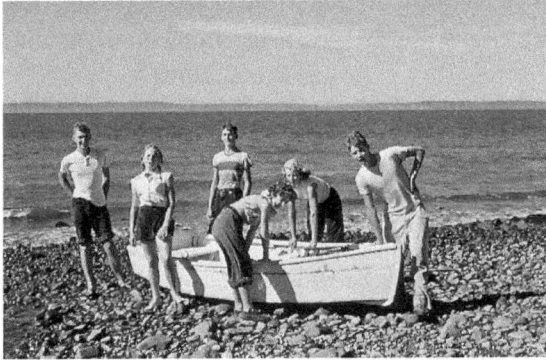

My Boat - L to R: me, Mary, Eric, Peggy, Elizabeth, Harold
Atwood Photo

A straight seasoned pole from one of the local weirs became the mast. Uncle Fred used his acetylene torch to cut an iron centreboard that pivoted up inside the boat, allowing it to remain upright when, at low tide, the harbour was empty of water. I obtained a pair of oars, had Fred Merritt "step" the mast and "rig" the sail. He insisted a marine compass should be installed permanently in the boat before it left the harbour. Any vessel that ventured out into the Bay of Fundy required one, he said, even my ten-foot dinghy. It could be needed to guide the way home if dense fog appeared, as it often did, without warning. The foghorn on the Isle of Haut, loud enough to be heard in certain atmospheric conditions over the mountain in the town of Berwick, could be muffled by the fog and become non-directional. If that happened, the fishermen would stop their boat engines and listen for the waves on the shore to help orient themselves. Their boats had foghorns to prevent collisions with each other. I decided to use my Scout whistle to serve as a foghorn to signal my presence on all my trips.

The currents associated with the tides were interesting. The rush of water up the bay created eddies with secondary currents of water going in the opposite direction closer to shore. These currents were stronger than the wind in our sails and could quickly pull our boat off course, but could also be used to speed us to our destination. The harbour at low tide was empty of water, the boats sitting on dry ground, unable to leave even if I needed to be rescued. My trial-and-error sailing lessons could only proceed within the harbour at full tide.

I stayed within the harbour until I too was shipshape and competent enough to go out into the ocean, captain of my own sailing yacht. I left the harbour each time with excitement and trepidation.

Paul Bishop, who was a childhood friend, and whose family had a cottage nearby, admired my boat. He borrowed my plans and constructed a sailing dinghy of his own. Soon we were sailing together out in the bay, giving rides to friends, siblings, and the Cogswell and Killam cousins, Margaret (Peggy) and Harold Atwood.

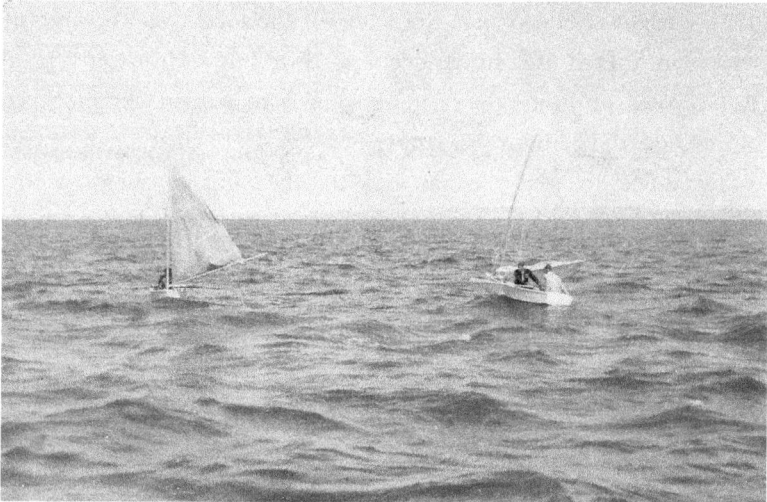

Paul and me in heavy winds.

I stayed near the wharf, but Paul was braver and was soon using the tides to sail to Black Rock, the next village. One day, when the winds and tides seemed perfect, I decided to brave the trip to Black Rock with Paul; we also took Peggy and Harold with us. Before we got back, the winds suddenly increased, and we heard the thunder that heralded a hurricane. We were anxious but managed to get back before those on land could send a rescue vessel.

There had been some concern around our ability as sailors. Later, at the cottage, Ora, the Cogswell/Killam/Atwood grandmother, suggested we record our adventure for posterity. She interrupted our games and insisted we do this in the guest book. I scribbled a couple of lines. Cousin Peggy, however, contributed something of lasting value. Her cartoon sketch of all of us sailing that day remains a valuable documentation of our family connections and of the fun we had together those many summers ago.

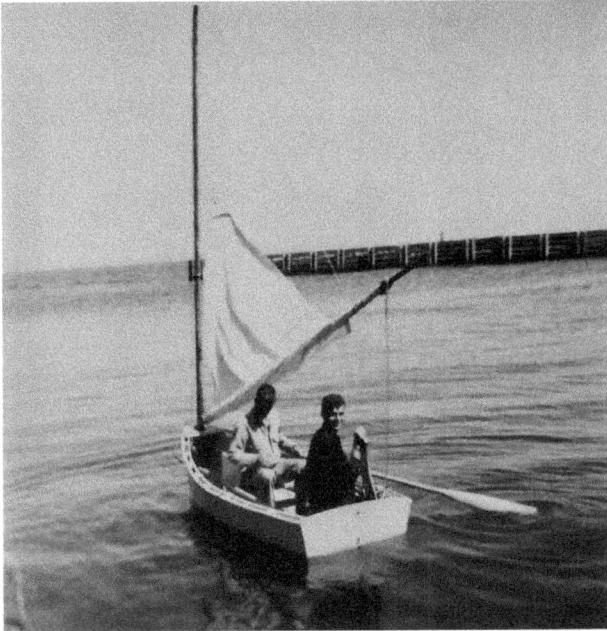

My cousin Harold and me in my boat—dubbed Weedoodit by my cousin Peggy (Margaret) Atwood—sailing off Harbourville harbour where my grandfather had a cottage.

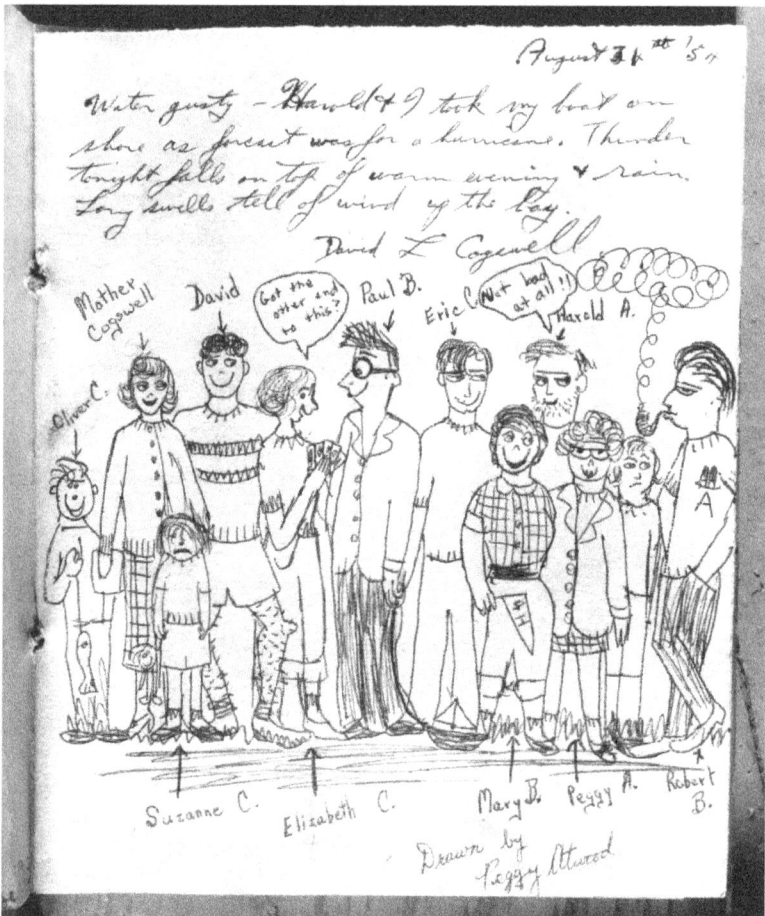

*My entry in the cottage log book describes taking the boat out on the Bay from
Harbourville. The illustration drawn by Margaret (Peggy) Atwood includes eight cousins,
my mother and three Bishop siblings. Back row from left to right: Oliver, Kathleen,
David, Elizabeth, Paul Bishop, Eric, Harold, and Robert Bishop; front row: Suzanne,
Mary Bishop, and Peggy herself. The smaller female on her right is my sister, Mary.
Picture included by kind permission of Margaret Atwood.*

The Making of
Country Doctors

I now wish I had asked my maternal grandfather Killam more about his early life, his childhood, his reasons for becoming a physician. I do know that prior to entering university he worked in a hardwood chair factory in the United States. He later taught school. Despite many of the students being his own age, he bragged there were no problems with discipline after they saw him casually lift a heavy dictionary using only the thumb and fifth finger of one hand. The class realized his strength, and no one wanted a confrontation. Savings from these jobs allowed him to enter the Halifax Medical College (later Dalhousie Medical School).

I know Grandfather had a sense of humour because one time he showed me a letter from Robert Ripley asking his permission to use his name, Doctor Harold Edwin Killam—or "Dr. He Killam"—in his *Ripley's Believe It or Not!* Grandfather had decided not to permit such "foolishness" but told me he could do even better. His best friend in medical school was Dr. Slaughter; his first nurse had been a Skinner; and many of his patients had been Eaton. He would add that in the local community, "hills" were described as "mountains": the hill in the west was the "North Mountain" and the one in the east, the "South Mountain." Sisters living in the area were "Brothers" even though their brothers were "Brothers" as well.

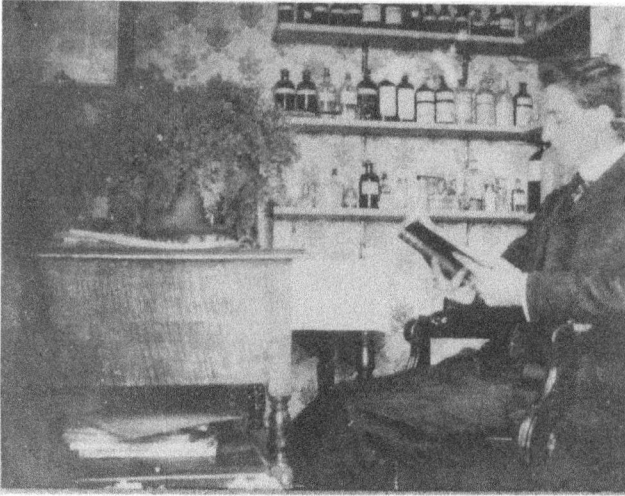

*My maternal grandfather, Dr. Harold E. Killam, on his first day in his home office
— Woodville*

I also know that when he returned home following his graduation as a doctor in 1906, Grandfather Killam was greeted at the
train station by a large contingent of the Woodville community who
begged him to stay and be their physician. Overcome by so much
support, he remained and practiced for the rest of his life in the
village where he grew up.

My father, Laverne, grew up on the Morristown family farm and
was ambivalent about farming. Eidson Cogswell, his father, did not
think farming a good occupation for his son and wanted him to
attend university. Laverne's dislike for managing farm animals was
amplified yearly when he hayed an isolated hot meadow with horse
and wagon. Alone, he cut hay with a scythe, raked and loaded it.
Ordering the horse forward, the cycle was repeated again and again.
The first thing Dad did after buying the farm from his father, Eidson,
was to sell the meadow and extend the orchards.

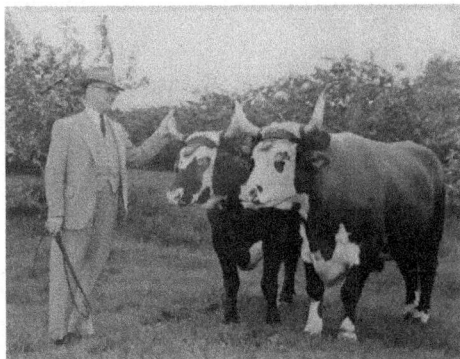

My father, Laverne, with oxen at family farm in Morristown.
Dave Thomas Photo

Dad's mother, Naomi Cogswell (Nichols), a schoolteacher, also encouraged him to enter university despite his severe dyslexia, a condition not well understood at the time. His hesitancy when reading caused some to consider him mentally "slow." When we were kids, he enjoyed reading to us, and we enjoyed his attention as we sat on his lap, but the stories took a long time. He read each letter out loud and then pronounced the word: "T-H-E . . . the . . . C-A-T . . . cat . . . I-S . . . the cat is . . . " and so on, until he had mastered the whole sentence. Despite this difficulty and the two-mile walk to a one-room school, he graduated and completed university. He suffered frequent headaches which he blamed on astigmatism. I think there was a tension component to them as well. He subsequently obtained a Bachelor of Science degree from Acadia and a medical degree from Dalhousie University.

I asked my father's advice prior to my applying for medical school. He recommended medicine as a rewarding occupation, where skills constantly improved with experience and better understanding of how patients responded to illness. He enjoyed helping people so much he continued working even after he became quite disabled. I believe my father, Laverne, was well suited as a country doctor.

I never considered any occupation other than medicine. I knew and had lived the lifestyle, as my father had his office in the house. From an early age I accompanied him on house calls and on hospital visits, where the matron-administrator, the nurses, even other physicians entertained me, while he made rounds.

Later when I was in practice, I took my own children to the WKMH, where they were welcomed, as once I had been. One of my children accompanied me for the drive to another hospital where I also had staff privileges but fewer patients. We received a hostile reception. The administrator informed me I would be reported to the board for bringing noise, distractions, and infections into the hospital. If this dangerous practice was repeated, she said, I would be expelled from staff. I received yet a different reception in a community 35 miles away from my home. A patient of mine attending the same banquet dropped a knife on her sandaled foot which required suturing. I gave her first aid and drove her to the local hospital where I was not on staff. We were informed that the doctor on call was busy with another emergency and would be for some time. My patient then revealed I was her family doctor, and the nurse suggested I do the repair. Once I had the laceration closed, the nurse turned to me and asked, "Who are you?", since she did not know me and needed to chart my name and I needed to record the procedure. Such different responses.

I did not enjoy my childhood trips with my father when he visited the local municipal chronic mental disease hospital. There I saw people walking in circles like animals within a ten-foot-tall wire caged-in area. They looked like prisoners. Even after I was told they were behind the fence for their own protection, to keep them safe, they still frightened me. Years later the introduction of anti-psychotic medications allowed many of these patients to return to their communities and the enclosed area disappeared. I was the local municipal hospital doctor during that period and was privileged to participate in these changes.

From an early age I accompanied my father to Valley Medical Society meetings[5], where I knew and was known by most of the doctors in the area. To officially become part of this medical fraternity, I needed to gain admission to medical school. Sixteen years old and in Grade 11, I had to choose how to continue my education. Grade 12 was not taught in Berwick, but I could complete my high school in either Kentville or Middleton. This would require me to board away from home for the school year. Or I could enter university, as Dalhousie University at that time admitted students with Grade 11 matriculation, and if I earned an optional high school Latin credit, I would be able to directly enter Dalhousie's Pre-Med program. I decided to add Latin to my Grade 11 studies, skip Grade 12, and enter Pre-Med at Dalhousie in the last class before it was extended from a two to a three-year program. This would save me a year of high school and a year of university.

Of the seven students attending my Berwick Grade 11 class, I was the only one requiring a Latin credit for university admission. The Latin classes were given after regular school hours, so it seemed like punishment. They became irregular due to teacher time conflicts, and finally were discontinued, leaving me unprepared to write the school final exam. I still had the summer to prepare for the fall university entrance exam. My summer vacation began with me studying at home, in the car in the driveway, the only quiet area I could find. My mother helped but became concerned by my slow progress and decided I had too little time to learn enough to pass. All her lessons ceased. My father, however, continued to encourage my study. He believed I could pass the entrance exam which would eliminate me needing to take a full first-year university Latin course. I kept working on my own.

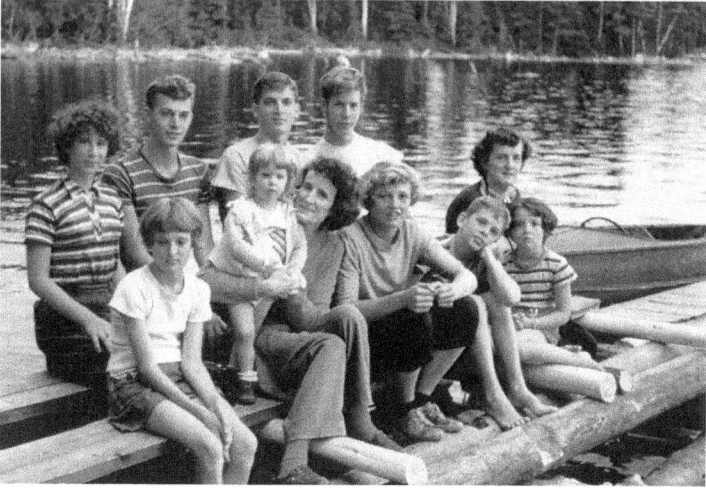

The Cogswell and Atwood families got together at Strawberry Island, Quebec, where Uncle Carl and Aunt Margaret had a camp. Back row left to right: Peggy Atwood, me, Eric Cogswell, Harold Atwood, Kathleen Cogswell (Mom). Front: Mary Cogswell (Graham), Ruth Atwood, Aunt Margaret Atwood, Elizabeth Cogswell (Pineo), Oliver Cogswell, Suzanne Cogswell.

My mother and her sister had planned a two-family two-week summer vacation to be spent at the Atwood's cottage in the Quebec wilderness, with Uncle Carl, Aunt Margaret, and cousins Harold and Peggy. My father stayed behind to work. Mother insisted I go, to share the driving. She believed I should enjoy the summer rather than spending my vacation studying for an examination I was likely to fail. Happy to have an excuse not to study, I went gladly, excited to be part of the wilderness camping. My exam preparation time now had shrunk by two weeks.

When we returned from our trip, Dad announced he had registered me for the exam while I was away enjoying myself with my cousins. He insisted I return to my studies and write the exam. I resumed my studies in the quiet and privacy of the parked car. The first thing I wrote on my examination paper was "Pre-Med" in large black print; I passed.

I entered university in Halifax that September. My mother arranged for my aunt Joyce Barkhouse to accommodate me within her family in Jollimore. Daily I crossed the Northwest Arm on a small ferry to attend classes and university activities in Halifax. I knew no one at the university, few in the city, and I remain grateful to this day to my aunt and her family for taking me into their home, grateful as well to my Bennet cousins who, hardly knowing me, opened their Halifax home and hearts to provide a haven in the city.

The Christmas physics examination shattered my hope of demonstrating I was capable of university. I grieved all the holidays thinking I had failed physics, but when I returned to university in January, I found I was third in the class. I informed my professor he must have made a mistake, for I had calculated the best I could have achieved was a maximum of 47. He told me the grades had been adjusted using a Bell Curve, something I did not understand. A week later my professor and the head of the department were waiting to speak to me as I left the class. They recommended I change my major from Pre-Med to Physics. Relieved, I understood I was university material and could be a doctor.

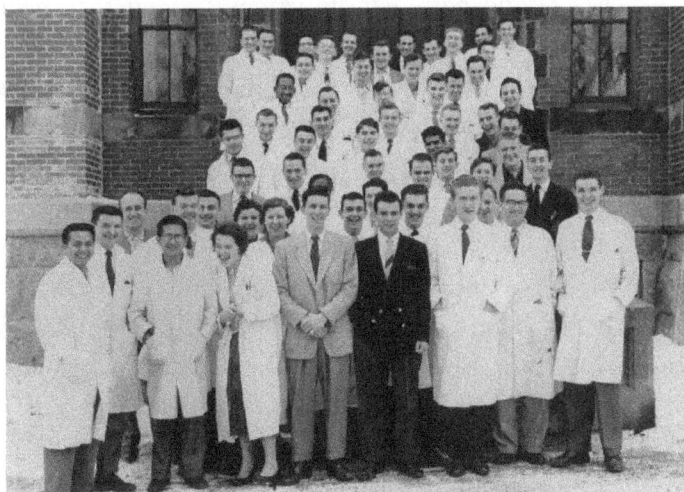

February 22, 1958 Dalhousie medical school class of 1960.
I am third from left in second to last row.

Two years rapidly passed, and I applied for medical school. To my surprise and horror, I was one of three Pre-Med students who had failed philosophy. Our applications to medicine were refused. Our professor had decided no one eighteen years or younger could be a philosopher. Lucky for all three of us a special supplemental exam was arranged by the university. We all passed. John MacKeigan, later an internal medicine specialist, made 50 percent; I made 51 percent; and Donald Hill, who became a pioneer in cardiac surgery, made 52 percent. We three were admitted to medical school and graduated together.

Following graduation in 1960, I was one of over 60 percent of the class who decided to specialize. The consultants had expected most of us would enter family medicine and were concerned when so many wanted to enter their specialties. I began my first year of surgical training in St. John's Newfoundland under Dr. G. Brownrigg, who was a very competent, considerate, and truly wonderful mentor. He was planning a new medical school in Newfoundland and encouraged me to return as a member of his staff when I completed my training. My second post-graduate year was in internal medicine at Camp Hill Hospital, Halifax. Shortly after my arrival, the nurse director told me the staff, because of my ability, were using me as the chief resident, bypassing the official senior resident.

The Dalhousie Department of Medicine had recently been reorganized by Torontonian Dr. Dickson into a cohesive, progressive service, and the University now began reorganizing its Department of Surgery. They recruited a surgeon from the British Health Service to develop and then head the department. The house staff were unimpressed by this man's surgical ability and irritating attitude and gave him the nickname "Zorro." The previously independent heads of each surgical subspecialty now became subservient to "Zorro"; they did not welcome these changes. Several excellent Halifax surgeons who had vied for the position and lost felt overlooked and unappreciated. They became less than cooperative. Naïvely unaware of this power struggle, I began the third year of my four-year training under "Dr. M," one of these disgruntled surgeons. It soon became apparent that I had more to learn from Dr. Bernard Steel, a recent graduate new to the service, than I did from Dr. M.

One morning, as we began abdominal procedure, Dr. M. told me to do the case; he would assist. I began with a new, more anatomical incision taught to me by Dr. Steele, which provided better access and less scarring than older more classical approaches. Dr. M became very angry, took over, and closed my incision. He then made the traditional incision and did the procedure himself.

A few weeks later, Dr. M. announced he would perform radical surgery on a ward patient who had returned with extensive spread of his disease despite several earlier radical surgical procedures. This would be the last surgery possible against the aggressive cancer. Dr. M. realized this deforming surgery would not be curative so he planned to insert a cannula in a local artery through which repeated injections of high levels of chemotherapy would be administrated, which might slow the spread of cancer not removed. These painful injections would then be continued for weeks following surgery. We were informed this procedure would be a world first, which Dr. M. planned to write up in a journal. At that time there were no hospital review or ethics committees. Surgery was booked for the following day. The house staff were told to get the permission. No one wanted to do it. Despite my initial refusal, as the newest resident I was compelled to go. The patient, who appeared dubious, asked if I would have it done on myself. I told him I would not. He refused to sign. Angry, Dr. M. never spoke to the patient to discuss the procedure with him, or request his permission, and surgery was cancelled.

Within the week I was summoned before "Zorro", now head of the Dalhousie Surgical Departments. With only the two of us in his office, keeping me standing, he remained officiously behind his desk. He told me he had it on good authority that I knew nothing, had learned nothing, had developed poor surgical techniques, and did not follow the instructions of my superiors. He would not give me any credit for the year, nor would he provide me any future references. I was shocked. I tried to give my side of what happened. "Zorro" would not listen. I then asked if he would consider taking me in his service and make his decision after working with me on the hospital wards and in the operating room. This he refused to do, but he added, almost as an afterthought, that he expected me to honour my contract and complete the last six months of my year's training. Encouraged, I asked if I would be able to redeem myself if I completed my year to his satisfaction. His reply: he would not change his mind no matter what I did. I wondered to myself, if he thought me so incompetent, why would he want me to continue treating his patients? I looked at him and asked if he thought I was crazy. "How stupid do you think me to be? I am a fully licensed physician in both Nova Scotia and Newfoundland with two years more documented training than any family physician in either province. I am qualified to practice anywhere in Canada. I have a wife, a two-year-old child, and we are expecting another, all of whom are dependent upon me. Surely you do not think I am so stupid as to remain in your control." I do not think he expected this of me, a twenty-six-year-old. I left, went directly to the hospital, picked up my belongings, and then went home to try to explain to my wife something that not even I could digest, understand, or believe had happened. I was too embarrassed to admit I had been fired to discuss it with anyone except immediate family. I was very fortunate to have a wife who was supportive.

I wonder to this day why none of the staff dared to intervene or even cared enough to call and offer me sympathy. I still am amazed that no one came to my defence. The only exception was Dr. Bernard Steele who, decades later, during the eight years we worked together as members of the provincial licensing authority, the Provincial Medical Board (PMB), privately took me aside to apologize for not speaking in my favour. He told me, at the time he was on probation himself and Dr. M. would have blocked his application for permanent staff membership. We were both bullied. Bullying is still occurring in medicine, as has been revealed in a recent article in the *Canadian Medical Association Journal* (*Lauren Vogel, December 10, 2018*). Patients are now protected by hospital ethics committees and courts have set legal precedent which were not available to me. Interestingly, following my dismissal, Dr. M. wrote an episode for the television series *Ben Casey*, about a rebellious resident who created havoc and could not be controlled by a junior staff man. An excellent senior doctor steps in and saves the day.

I needed to be able to protect myself and my medical licence. If the head of surgery really believed me incompetent, he would be legally and morally responsible to ask the Provincial Medical Board (PMB)) to revoke my licence. I contacted both Dr. G. Brownrigg and Dr. R. M. McDonald, my previous mentors, and explained my predicament. Both offered to provide good references if needed for the PMB, or for any future resident training applications I might make. No longer wanting to be a surgeon, or deal with them, I decided to become an ophthalmologist, a specialty that would combine my interests in physics and surgery. I applied to the University of Toronto's Eye Course, one of the best in Canada. I had good interviews, but their positions for the coming year were filled.

My immediate need was to support my family, until I could reapply for ophthalmology the following year. I began searching for a general practice position in either Newfoundland or Nova Scotia. A clinic in an affluent area of Dartmouth offered me a position as a junior member. I realized this city practice would provide immediate income but not the independence and variety both my father and grandfather enjoyed all their lives in their country practices. My surgical training would be wasted. The monotony and stress of an urban practice had some of these doctors looking at other medical fields, or planning early retirement, which contrasted greatly with the experiences of both my grandfather and father, neither of whom had even considered retirement.

I knew grandfather loved practicing rural medicine and had been interested in the changes and advancements in treatment, incorporating them into his practice. Illness had forced him to close his practice years before I began med school but he maintained his interest. He described treating pneumonia in the pre-antibiotic era, the patient developed a dramatic rise in temperature over a twenty-four to forty-eight-hour period, then its sudden fall (the "crisis"). Lacking modern antibiotics, he could only treat symptoms and could predict which patient would live or die. Reading his *Osler Textbook of Medicine,* I realized bleeding was still listed as a treatment for pneumonia when he trained, one I doubt he ever utilized. Medical therapy had advanced greatly during his practice years. He then surprised me, asking me not to discuss anything connected with medicine. He told me he loved general practice so much his sleep was disturbed nightly by dreams he was still working. The more he discussed medicine, the more vivid were his dreams.

I felt capable to begin country family practice. I had given anaesthetics while interning and while doing a locum. Aylesford needed a physician, and I had a family to feed. I started a solo practice, working closely with my father and Dr. Paul Kinsman[6]. Although I worked very hard, I made little money. Patients unable to pay or who owed other physicians came to "Dr. David." Shortly after the birth of our second child in March of 1963, I received a letter from the University of Toronto informing me that I would be accepted the following year in ophthalmology if I applied. I considered my situation. I had already spent three years doing my surgical training. Ophthalmology would entail three more years, during which family time would continue to suffer. My oldest would be in school and I would have missed her childhood. My wife would have been left to bring up the family alone. My father, who had MS, was now relying on me. I had no financial reserves. I was needed in the community. I liked what I was doing. I decided not to apply; I was now a country doctor.

Father and Grandfather's Practice

My father was a family physician whose office was an integral part of our house. Patients entered his office through a common vestibule containing two inside doors, one giving access to his office, the other to our kitchen. The small vestibule with seating for four became the waiting area. His patients and practice were always an intimate part of our home life. There were no appointments, no secretary, no proper waiting room. The office consisted of one room with a desk, sink, and examining table. The room had an L-shaped extension, its three walls lined floor to ceiling with shelves full of the medications he dispensed. We children were allowed to go in the office but prohibited to go near the bottles of pills and liquids.

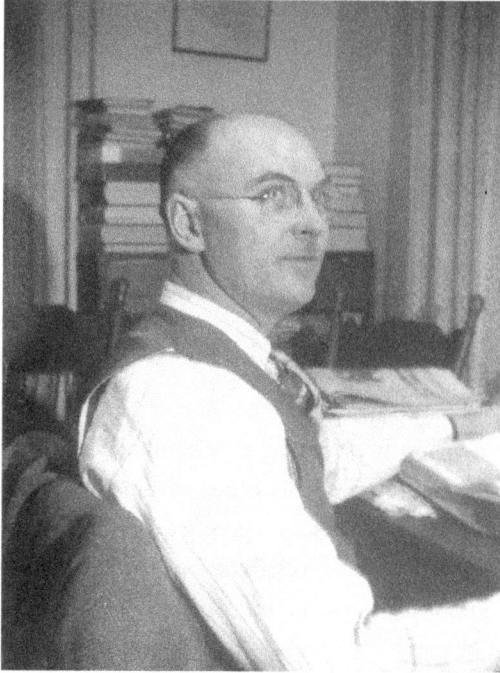

Dr. Laverne Cogswell in office
David Cogswell

To manage alone, Dad had developed many shortcuts. If he was away on house calls, Mother answered the door, the phone, and sold the medications he had assembled. She did this in addition to caring for the house and six children. She seemed to know each patient, and on occasion would refill prescriptions herself, always keeping a record for my father. If both of my parents were away, I would collect the $1.50 or $2.00 written on the small box and give out the drugs. On one occasion a patient browbeat me to fill his empty pillbox when my parents were not at home. He helped by showing me where dad kept the stock bottle. I was severely reprimanded when my parents returned. I was not to dispense drugs.

ster

BERWICK NS CANADA
HOP 1E0 02/01/2001

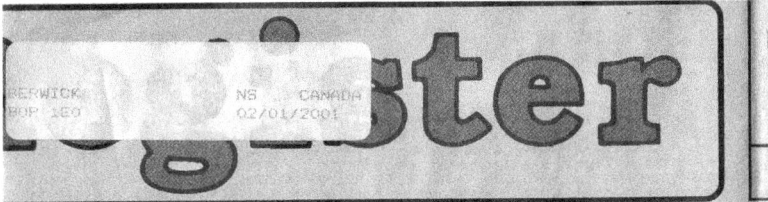

ible people highlight of country doctor

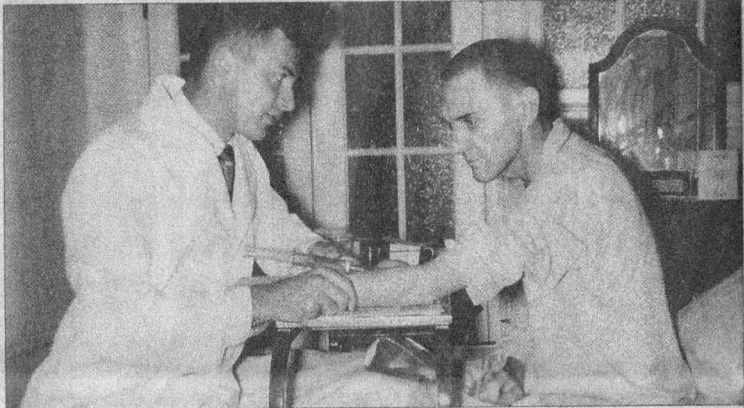

Young Dr. David Cogswell, left, spent time early in his career of general medicine at the Nova Scotia Sanatorium in Kentville, helping patients there with TB and asthma conditions. Now, almost 40 years later, Dr. Cogswell has retired from a successful community practice in Aylesford. A lot has changed in that time.   (Submitted)

Me while at Nova Scotia Sanatorium (1959)
Berwick Register

From an early age I assisted in the office, holding Dad's instruments while he sutured, or steadying heads for tooth extractions. When I was home from medical school, he would call me to the office to see interesting cases and taught me some office procedures. One patient with severe asthma suggested that under Dad's supervision I give him the intravenous aminophylline occasionally required to control acute flare-ups of his disease. Learning to enter a vein with a needle and how to administer the medicine would be a good learning experience for me, a new skill, this patient decided, and he allowed me to give him the medicine on several occasions. One day he appeared at the office severely distressed. My father was away, the patient was deteriorating and begging me to give him the medication, which I did. His breathing returned to normal. I kept him there for my father to review on his return. I was not reprimanded.

A few months later I was a Junior Intern at the Nova Scotia Sanitorium in Kentville when the local paper ran a feature detailing the evolving role of the Sanitorium with the rapid improvements in the treatment of Tuberculosis. There was an inpatient in the San who required the same medication I had given my father's patient, and our picture was used to headline the article.

Our kitchen mirror was carefully mounted and angled to allow Dad to see by reflection any and all who entered the office door. His dining room chair was strategically placed and with a slight movement he could make himself invisible to anyone who might, in turn, see his reflection. "Come in and sit down, (Tom…Jane,) and I'll be with you as soon as I have finished my dinner," was his standard welcome to patients who came at mealtime.

My mother was used to the practice of medicine invading the home. During her childhood, her father also worked from a home office, which was the norm for most country doctors of that era. These home offices were convenient for both the physician and the community. All knew where the doctor lived and would appear with their illnesses and injuries at almost any time of the day or night.

Anxious to spend time with our busy father, we children frequently accompanied him on house calls, even going with him to the hospital, where the nurses entertained us while he visited patients. Intuitively, I knew from an early age that medical care was a personal thing provided in the office, the hospital, or in patients' homes, wherever the best, most effective and convenient care could be provided. Rural physicians often consulted one another but more formal consultations required a trip to Halifax. Even in good weather, these trips could be difficult and long. Uncle Fred, Mother's brother, remembered a trip home in a dense fog, driving with his head stuck out of the window, following telephone poles, hoping for glimpses of the road. He was fortunate to be able to follow the headlights of a car whose driver seemed to know the road. Suddenly the guiding lights of the car in front of him stopped moving. Fred made an emergency stop and walked indignantly forward to chastise the driver. Only then did he realize the car was neatly parked in its own garage.

My father had a very large practice, most of whom were fearful of the drive to the city, and who had no financial resources. Lacking urban knowledge, once there, they would be unable to find their way to the doctors' offices. Frequently my father made their Halifax appointment, took them in his own car to the consultant, waited for them and brought them back home. If there were any patients from his practice in a Halifax hospital, he visited them while he was waiting.

He was obviously upset one evening after a busy office. He had seen an infant that was failing to thrive and had learned the mother was feeding the child flour and water. She told him it looked like the milk she could not afford. He provided the proper infant formula for the child and told her to return for more as it was needed. He told her it was from a supply of samples he had received and more would be coming. I am sure he gave out many of these "samples" to needy patients.

Living in their midst and hearing stories from my father and my grandfather about their professional lives influenced me long before I began medical school. I followed naturally in their footsteps, assuming from childhood I would be a doctor.

My grandfather's stories often included a reference to Gem, his favorite horse and reflected his love of country medical practice. They mostly began "in the winter of the deep snow . . ." This was the term used by many of his generation who remembered that particularly difficult year. I never did learn the exact date to which he referred, but it must have been in the decade between 1910-20. Bridges at that time were made as simply as possible, designed to go straight across the rivers. Most were narrow, one way, their approach at sharp angles to the road; there were frequent accidents, one of which grandfather remembered. A car had missed a bridge and gone into the river. When asked what had happened, the inebriated driver said he had seen the bridge coming down the road and pulled out to pass it. In addition to bridge design and alcohol, winding irregular roads and drifting snow all conspired to cause accidents in the same areas each winter. Everyone knew where fences would be taken down to allow sleighs access to open fields to circumvent these obstacles.

One day I commented to Grandfather that the Isle Haute (an island in the Bay of Fundy) seemed to have floated up the bay closer to Harbourville. He agreed that the island appeared at times to float up or down the Bay, and we decided certain atmospheric conditions conspired to make this mirage-like illusion. He went on to speculate the apparent changes in the position of the island might be the origin of the Mi'kmaq legend, describing it as "Glooscap's canoe." Then began the story of one of the winter trips with Gem.

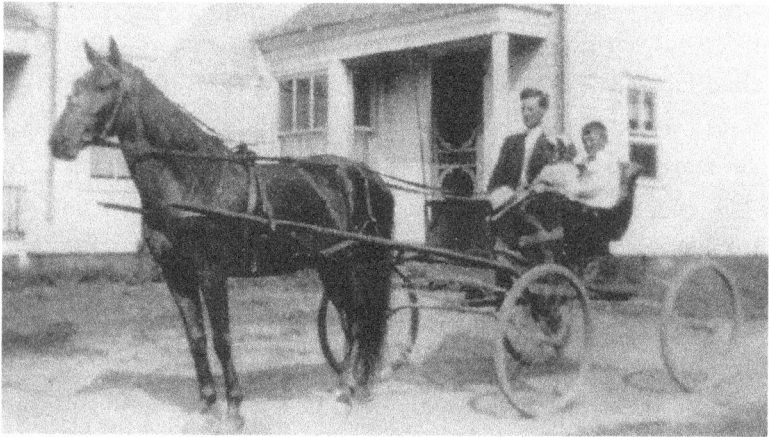

Dr. Harold E. Killam and his beloved horse, Gem, shown with two children.

Following the delivery of a young mother of her first baby, my grandfather was coming home from "over the mountain" in his sleigh. It was during "the winter of the deep snow." Wrapped in a buffalo robe against the severe cold, snow falling heavily all around, he was happy to be going home to bed. In the howling wind and the darkness, the view blocked by high snowbanks, he had difficulty being sure of his exact location. At each intersection he looked out into the Bay and rechecked his position using Isle Haute as a landmark. He knew the name of every road in the area, and although he could not see beyond the driving snow and the snowbanks, the island continued to guide and reassure him. After a time, he came to a crossroad where Gem wanted to head to the right. He checked their position with relation to the island, realized the horse wanted to go in the wrong direction, and urged her on to the proper road. With Gem bravely battling the weather they came to another crossroad. Again, Gem wanted to go to the right. He looked out at the island and urged Gem on to the correct road. A third intersection appeared where Gem wanted to go in one direction and he in another. Suddenly he realized he was at the same corner for the third time. He was going in circles. Lost and cold, both he and the horse were tired. He carefully checked their position with that of the island. It was still obvious that Gem wanted to go in the wrong direction. He, however, realized his navigation had thus far taken them in circles, and they were now lost. In desperation, he let the horse take her own lead. She took the other road, the road that seemed incorrect, and went straight home. My grandfather credited Gem with saving both their lives that winter night.

On another occasion, again following a long sleepless night managing a home birth, Gem was taking Grandfather home while he slept in the buggy. Gem could be relied upon to find her way home without any direction from him. Suddenly he was jolted awake. Someone had run out from their house and had grabbed Gem's bridle and stopped the buggy. The man holding the bridal was one of a few in the area to have a new device: a telephone. Grandfather was needed for an emergency back at the house where he had just completed the delivery. It was common knowledge which household in each small community had a phone. The family with the newborn baby had guessed how far Grandfather and his horse had progressed and contacted the nearest home by phone, requesting they have the doctor return. Fearing that either something had gone wrong with the newborn baby, or that the new mother was having a post-partum haemorrhage, Grandfather turned the wagon around and rushed back. His anxiety for the new mother and child had erased his tiredness.

When he arrived at the home, he was astonished to find the father was the emergency. In his excitement about being the father of a healthy child and the husband of a healthy wife, he had accidently grabbed the blade of the scythe he was sharpening. By so doing, he had deeply lacerated his palm and severed most of the flexor tendons of his hand. Grandfather knew the wound needed to be repaired urgently. The nearest surgeon and hospital were in Halifax, days away. One Halifax surgeon came monthly on the morning train to the valley, operated all day, and then boarded the train on its evening return to Halifax, leaving the post-operative care to the local physicians—but this visit was weeks away. The hand could not wait that long. Grandfather would have to do the repair in the home. The reality of country medical practice of his day was that most solo physicians, at one time or another, were forced to use unorthodox methods to deal with emergencies. This was one of those kitchen table operations.

As was his custom, and that of most rural physicians when attending home deliveries, he carried an obstetrical kit containing chloroform, ether, sutures, and instruments, in addition to his regular medical bag. Grandfather now needed a member of the household to administer the anaesthetic. Despite the assurance he would continuously direct and monitor any volunteers, all adamantly refused. They were either squeamish or too afraid. Grandfather had no choice; he would have to do both—give the anaesthetic and do the surgery himself.

Grandfather had an excellent knowledge of anatomy. He well knew the mid-palmer area of the hand was known as "no man's land" by surgeons, as most repairs of severed flexor tendons in that area do poorly. The proximal end of the tendon retracts into its sheath, is difficult to grasp, and the bulge produced by the repair inhibits its movement within the tight flexor sheath.

With all his sutures and instruments ready, Grandfather put the patient to sleep, deeply asleep. Then began the repair, working as fast as he could until the anaesthetic began to wear off. At that point he administered more of the anaesthetic agent, again producing a deep sleep. He continued this process of working between the sterile and unsterile areas, alternatively becoming the anesthesiologist, then the surgeon, until the repair was completed.

The patient moved away shortly after, and contact was lost. Over the years the episode was forgotten. During one of my frequent visits home from medical school, Grandfather was eager to tell me some interesting news. The man whose hand he had repaired years before had come unannounced to the door. Grandfather feared he had come to show him an unusable hand. But the patient had come to show him an almost perfect hand, and to thank him.

It is strange how history repeats itself. I had a somewhat similar experience that affected me in the same way. I had been in practice for many years when my secretary told me she had booked a new patient. I was surprised, as I was not accepting new patients. She said that this man had been so insistent she had relented, and he was here for his appointment. I started the interview by asking about his past health. He immediately informed me he was not there as a patient but had come for two reasons: the first was to thank me; the other was to pay the bill his mother must still owe me. Reviewing his name and that of his mother, I began remembering this family.

Years before, when the man was a child, his mother had come to my office with her children. She was a single parent who lived "over the mountain." Although they were warmly dressed, their clean clothes were somewhat worn. The children were well-behaved and cooperative. As they had come by taxi, I assumed they had some type of financial support and gave them prescriptions to fill at the drug store. I continued to provide care for other illnesses following that initial visit.

Around midnight one evening I received a phone call from a woman who said she was a neighbour of theirs. The eldest child, now the man before me, was at her door asking her to take his very sick sibling to the doctor. She informed me the family lived in a small run-down house in a field behind her home, without a car or telephone. It was snowing so heavily, the caller did not dare drive down the mountain to my office, for fear she might be unable to get home again.

As was my practice, I made the requested home visit. After examining the child, I provided the mother with enough sample medications to treat the illness. When asked why she had not called me earlier about the child's illness, she admitted to a lack of money for a taxi or medications. I urged her in the future to call me whenever she or the children were sick, and I would come to her home bringing medical samples. There would be no charge. After a few years they had left the area. Now the son was here to pay his mother's bill and to thank me. I was overwhelmed. No one had ever come to pay such a bill. I thanked him for coming and told him there had never been a bill, once I was aware of the family's finances. I had been pleased to care for the family, and his coming to thank me was more than enough payment.

Office Procedures

My grandfather dispensed drugs, which was the custom of most rural Nova Scotian physicians in 1906. In a photograph taken on his first day in practice, medications are proudly displayed on the wall behind his desk. I have the mortar and pestle that he used to compound his mixtures. There was no local pharmacy and doctors were known as much for their medications as for their diagnostic abilities. Grandfather indignantly remembered a patient complaining that the cough medicine he received was "no good," as the cough had continued following the office visit, even though he had drained the bottle before he reached the corner on the way home. I also have a small medical bag my grandfather used to carry his diagnostic equipment. He must have had other bags ready to take to home births, surgical emergencies, and other specific uses.

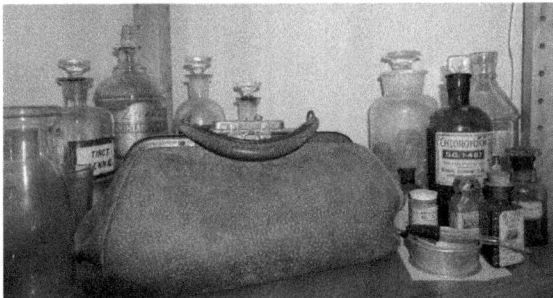

Dr. Harold Edwin Killam's Medical Bag
Cogswell Photo.

My father dispensed medications from a recessed area of his office where they were not visible to his patients but were immediately accessible. The two doors providing access to the office were never locked. We six children knew we were not allowed into any area of the office unless Dad was there. He continued to dispense even after two pharmacies opened in town. Dad had a large bag full of glass bottles of medications which accompanied him on house calls. Even if he had to walk through unplowed snow, it went with him; it weighed forty pounds. This enabled the sick to begin treatment immediately, without the added delay and expense of a trip to town to fill a prescription. Those who were financially unable to pay were not billed. Dad had a third bag, prepared and ready for home deliveries.

I remember accompanying him to visit a patient he had delivered. She had had a retained placenta that he had removed manually in her home as an emergency, to control bleeding, and he was checking her daily. She looked very pale to me, but he was pleased with her progress. I am amazed at the number of skills he had developed which enabled him to do so many home deliveries.

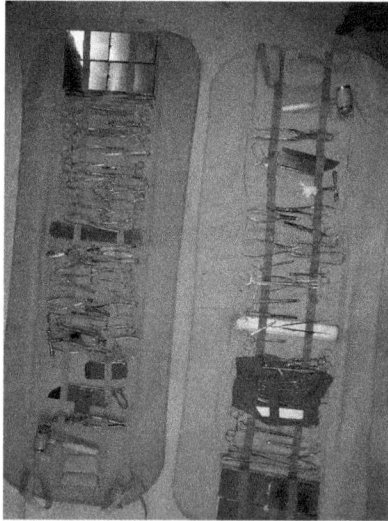

Contents of Dr. H.E. Killam's Field Medical Bag

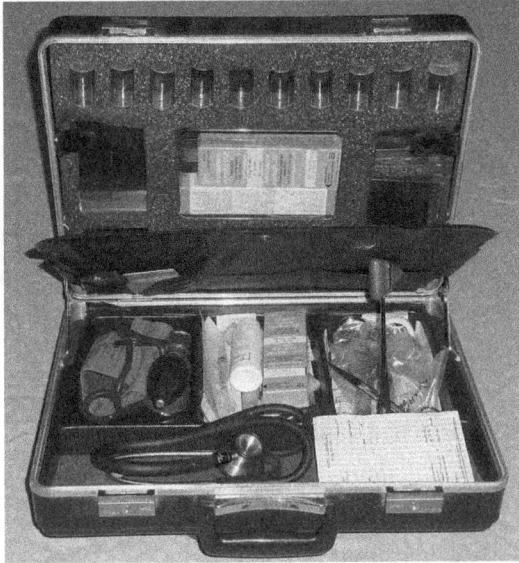

My medical bag with divider functioning as a writing surface.
Cogswell photo

When I began practice, I decided not to dispense drugs. When making house calls, I was able to provide my patients with their first twenty-four hours of medication using free samples left me by drug company representatives. Therapy begun, they were able to fill their prescriptions at a pharmacy at their convenience, and I gave enough samples to those unable to purchase medications to treat their illnesses. My medical bag contained diagnostic equipment, emergency inject-ables, and my laryngoscope as well as the drug samples. In a separate bag I carried face masks, endotracheal tubes and other ventilator resuscita-tive equipment which I always had with me—equipment not available to my predecessors. I did not need an obstetrical bag, for, unlike my father and grandfather, I did not plan to do home deliveries as a routine feature of my practice. The home births I did attend were unexpected emergencies, and at such times I borrowed hospital equipment.

All three generations of us managed minor wounds in our offices. We had instruments, sutures, needles that were sanitized using chemical baths and boiling water sterilizers. Disposable syringes and needles had not yet been invented, so our glass syringes needed to be carefully inspected and cleaned. The needles, in addition to careful cleaning, usually required sharpening on a fine whetstone. The sharper the needle, the less discomfort for the patient. We were grateful when the hospital outpatient department became available to us to do our more difficult suturing there, and for the invention of disposable syringes and needles.

When grandfather began his practice in 1906 there were no local hospitals. Kitchen table operations that required a colleague to assist had to be planned days ahead, or alternatively sent to a Halifax hospital. With the onset of World War 1 (WW1) in 1914, Grandfather Killam voluntarily enlisted in the army as a physician for Aldershot Camp and was issued a Field Surgery Kit, which is still in my possession.

It consisted of a canvas roll up bag, with his name, "H. E. KILLAM" inked on the outside. The kit was filled with a multitude of surgical instruments, each carefully secured. Many instruments are missing but their outline remains. The wide range of instruments in the kit reveals the variety of casualties a battlefield doctor was expected to encounter and treat. There were tools to remove bullets and shrapnel, although without the availability of X-rays, many fragments were missed. There were bone saws for amputations, multiple sutures and needles, even a tool to repair severed loops of bowel. Although he never served in a battlefield, Grandfather's kit appears well-worn. He must have been grateful to have these tools and equipment with him when he arrived in Halifax to treat victims of the 1917 Explosion. The city, at that horrific time, would have been like a huge battlefield.

Harold Edwin Killam & the Halifax Explosion 1917

Our Sundays began with Sunday school, then church. Following the noon meal, we visited the Killam grandparents. Upon arrival there, we were warned to "keep the noise down," as grandfather was having his nap. Then we were free to explore the children's closet full of mysterious playthings. One day we found, hidden behind the other toys, a make-believe rifle made of varnished wood cut crudely to the size and outline of a real gun. We were delighted. We knew grandfather hated guns, but this must have been one of his childhood toys. When he saw us marching, he admonished us. "Guns are not children's toys," he said, and it disappeared. Later we were told this had been his wartime "gun, "issued to him for his basic training so he would know how to march and maneuver a real gun, when one became available. Soldiers deployed overseas had been given all the existing rifles and the production of new weapons had not yet caught up to the demand. He was pleased that medical personnel had a low priority for guns and that the wooden one had remained his only gun, even after the occurrence of the Halifax Explosion.

Kentville received early knowledge of the Explosion perhaps because Aldershot military Camp was located there. The rumours in Halifax were that the explosion was part of a German invasion. George Graham walked from North Street Train Station in the city, to the first station left intact, which was in Rockingham. From there he was able to send telegrams to Kentville and other outside areas with information about the disaster and requesting help.

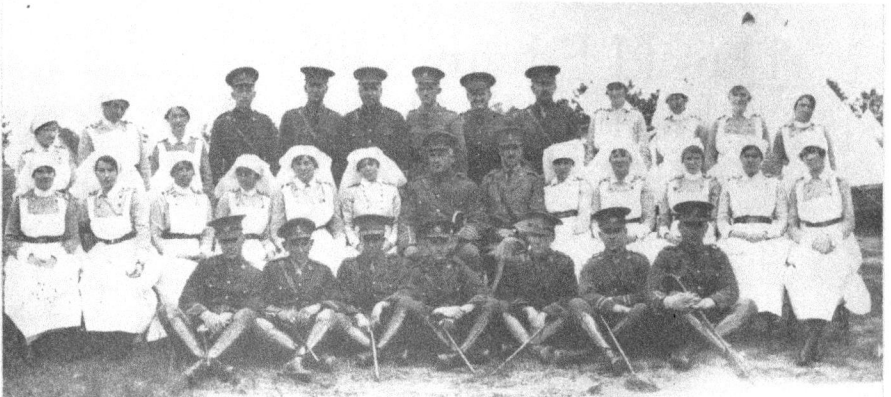

STAFF FIELD HOSPITAL, ALDERSHOT CAMP

Staff field hospital, Aldershot Camp with Dr. H.E. Killam.

Grandfather Killam was on the first relief train from Kentville. He had graduated in 1906, and to do his part in the war effort had joined the Army as a staff doctor at Aldershot Camp, while maintaining his Woodville practice at night and on weekends. My mother remembers watching her mother, Ora, helping him pack for Halifax. She added to his personal things any clothing in the house that could be spared. This was the only time Kathleen, my mother, saw her mother cry. Grandmother and Grandfather Killam were devastated by the news of the explosion and were especially concerned as Grandfather's brother Fred Killam owned a flower nursery in Halifax on Kay street overlooking the narrows where the ships collided.

Dr. Perc McGrath was on the same train. Later, when I was working with Perc, he gave me a copy of his photo of the "STAFF FIELD HOSPITAL, ALDERSHOT" medical team. When they arrived in Halifax, they worked at the Halifax Military Hospital on Cogswell Street.

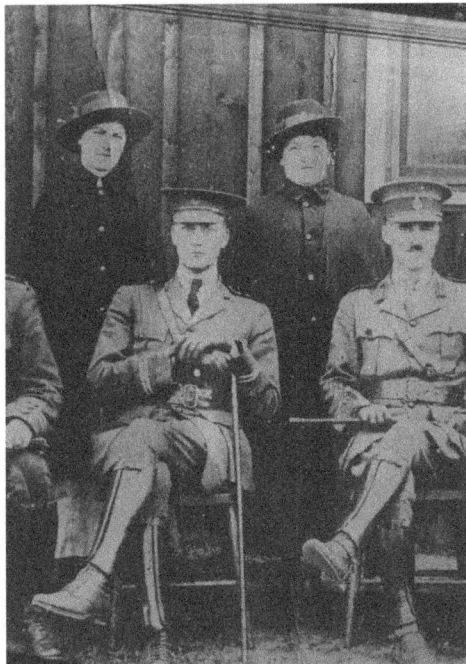

Dr. H.E. Killam on Left at Camp Aldershot during First World War

The picture includes Capt. H. E. Killam, Lt. J. P. McGrath, and Dr. W. W. Woodbury (later my orthodontist). Perc did not formally graduate from medicine until December 12th, 1917. I still have both the picture of the Aldershot Field Hospital staff given me by Perc, and the military medical kit[7] used by grandfather.

The explosion had destroyed the railway tracks, and only trucks could navigate the damaged roads leading into the city. Grandfather, admitting he knew it was a stupid question, asked the driver of the truck taking him into the city if knew his brother, Fred Killam, who owned a nursery. The driver not only knew Fred, but he also knew all members of the family had survived. What a relief! He later learned that when the explosion occurred, Fred had been sick in bed upstairs in his home on Kay Street. The house overlooked the narrows where the ships collided. The force of the explosion had carried him out of the destroyed home and landed him unhurt on the ground, still on his mattress. I remember his wife, Aunt Rose, as a plump woman. She had fallen two storeys into the basement. Looking up, she realized the opening in the floor above her where the staircase had been, and her only avenue of escape, was closing. She reached up, grabbed the sides, and pulled herself up to freedom. Her only obvious injury was bruising of her legs caused by the shrinking escape opening. Unfortunately, she later suffered a spontaneous miscarriage of the male child she was carrying.

Although the family survived, they were unable to rescue their horse from the burning barn.

Knowing his brother Fred Killam and family had survived Grandfather continued with the Aldershot Field Hospital staff to the Cogswell Street Military Hospital where I assume the team worked as a unit.

Antique Rolls-Royce & Antique Clock

I have always been interested in motor vehicles. My mother remembered, with amusement, that my first word was not "Mama" or "Papa," but "car." This lifelong car fever was stimulated during my preteen years by the rumour that somewhere in Annapolis County was a mystery Rolls-Royce, in which a man had been shot and killed. There were wildly different accounts suggesting why he had been murdered, who he might be, and where the car was located. All accounts acknowledged the existence of the Rolls Royce. They also agreed that in Annapolis county there was a widow living a solitary existence in a house with a Rolls Royce in show room condition, perfect except for a bullet hole, hidden in a bricked in enclosure in the basement of her house, placed there as a memorial to the man killed in it. The bullet-scarred Rolls had yet to be found.

Years later while helping Jim Patterson, an accomplished antique car restoration expert, rebuild my 1923 Dodge Brothers touring car, I brought up the Rolls story and suggested we go to Annapolis to find it. He laughed and told me that the story had already inspired him to search for the vehicle, as had many other collectors over the years. No such car had ever been found and he was now certain the car had never existed—it was only an interesting urban myth.

Sadly, about that time my great-aunt Lola Nichols died, bequeathing me her kitchen clock. She had always loved giving presents.

Christmas was her favourite time of the year. Her modest teacher's pension forced her to begin careful shopping for her many friends and family during the Boxing Day sales, and she continued shopping all year long. She wrapped each gift as it was found and added it to her Christmas pile. At any moment she immediately knew those for whom she had presents and those for whom she had yet to buy. Her last gift to me was this old clock she had instructed her family to give me following her death. It was intended as a memento of our times together, as none of my childhood visits to her Nicholsville home had been complete until we had viewed the moose-head trophy mounted in the front hall and the clock with the wooden mechanism on the kitchen wall. Little did I realize my love of the old clock would now lead me to an old car.

The clock was badly in need of repair when I received it—no longer working and with many layers of paint defacing it. Aunt Lo told me the routine when redecorating the kitchen had been to coat the clock and kitchen walls with the same paint, blending the two, but this had completely destroyed the original finish of the clock.

Opening the clock face revealed the original printed information sheet glued inside, announcing that "Roman M. Butler and Company" of Annapolis, Nova Scotia, was the manufacturer. Accompanying this information was a great deal of scribbled handwriting, the most intriguing of which was a list of dates from 1778 to 1786. Who had valued those dates enough to insert them on the inside of the most visible clock in the house, possibly the only clock they owned? Could the clock have been constructed in the 1770s? Were these dates an early maintenance record, and why were they there at all?

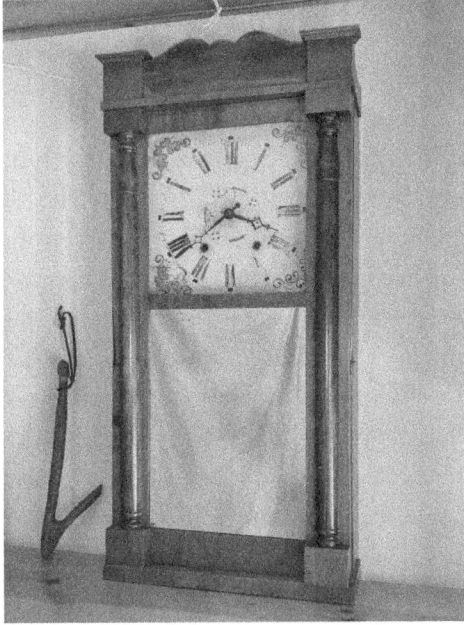

Nichols Family Clock with wooden mechanism, and Abner's Hook for holding apple basket

My mind began to wander . . . 1778, two years after the American rebels declared their independence from Britain. Many loyal citizens had escaped north to Nova Scotia as United Empire Loyalists. My Nichols ancestors were among this group; I knew this from family lore. The first to arrive was a pregnant widow who, with her son, had narrowly escaped capture. Her husband was not so fortunate. William Nichols had escaped capture and was fearful of being executed. In an attempt to get to Loyalist held territory he swam across the cold Delaware River, which contained ice flows. Only to be re-captured, he died a cruel death on the streets of Philadelphia. With a cry of, "If you are not with us, you are against us," he was cruelly ridden on a rail until he died.

Possibly this innocent widow, on her arrival in Annapolis, had been tempted by the wily Annapolis clockmaker to buy the clock. She would not have known the unscrupulous tricks the American salespeople often used, later depicted by Thomas Haliburton in his "Sam Slick" stories[8]. No matter, the clock that had been part of the Nichols household in Nicholsville for so many years was now mine and it needed restoration.

I learned of Norman Phinney, a retired Halifax musical instrument storeowner now living in Middleton, who collected and repaired clocks as a hobby, including those with wooden mechanisms. He kindly agreed to repair mine. His large collection of antique clocks is now owned by the Nova Scotia Museum, and part of this is also the main exhibit at the MacDonald Museum in Middleton. He told me he owned a clock like mine. It was by the same maker, with the original gold leaf finish intact. It had appeared garish to him when he viewed it under artificial light, but when he used period lighting with candles it glowed beautifully.

Apparently, the wooden clock mechanisms of the type in my clock had been developed to fill a need left by British clockmakers, who had been unable to obtain bronze to make their clocks. During the turbulent 1800s, bronze had been requisitioned by the British military and none was left for clock mechanisms. Resourceful Yankees had then developed wooden gears. The handwritten dates from 1778 preceded the manufacture of the clock itself. My romantic vision of the clock's history was dashed.

The clock restoration was begun by Hayden Woodworking in Berwick, who refinished the case. That done, Norman repaired the wooden mechanism. Three of the wheel gears were missing teeth sheared along the wood grain, a common occurrence. Norman replaced these teeth with diamond-shaped pieces of wood carefully inserted with the grain at ninety degrees to that of the wheel. These repaired gears were stronger than the originals. While working on the gears, Norman noticed the movement was the dirtiest he had ever seen. Cleaning off the waxy dirt to facilitate the customary oiling of the wire axles, he realised the dirt smelled of, and was, beeswax. Moreover, there was almost no wear on the surrounding wood and none of the usual oil-induced wood rot. Beeswax seemed a much better lubricant than oil. He carefully replaced the wax he had earlier removed and, now understanding its usefulness, added beeswax to his toolbox. It is interesting that Aunt Lo always emphasised to me not to use oil, only beeswax, as a lubricant for the wooden movement.

Norman noticed my 1965 American Rambler convertible and soon we were talking old cars as well, as old clocks. He began telling me about a woman who had arrived at his home from Annapolis Royal in a chauffeured car. She had brought with her an antique clock needing repair. She was so pleased when she saw her clock working, she returned with another even better clock for repair. The arrival of a third, even nicer clock so intrigued Norman that he decided to return this clock himself, hoping for a visit with the owner.

His hope materialized. Norman and his wife were invited in for tea; this began a new friendship. About a week following one of their subsequent visits, Norman received a call inviting him to return, as she had something she wanted to show him.

Roger, Norman's son, accompanied his father on this exciting occasion and remembers following their hostess down a ten-foot-wide corridor to a carpet-covered end wall. The carpet, when pulled aside, revealed a hidden door, which opened into a large storage area without any other means of access. Buried under a bed spring and other stored items, they were astonished to see the tattered remnants of a white, Limited Edition 1920 Rolls-Royce Silver Ghost automobile.

He later learned this was one of only two Rolls ever built in that body style; the other had gone to Australia. Despite being badly deteriorated, there was no bullet hole. It needed a complete rebuild, which would be labour intensive and require many replacement parts. Norman was delighted to see such a rare vehicle. He immediately realized this unusual classic car, following a careful restoration, would become a rare masterpiece. He offered to buy the Rolls, but his hostess refused to sell. She in all probability had never intended to sell the car and had hidden it to stop the stream of passers-by who came to her door asking about it. She now realized Norman's love of cars matched his love of clocks. She had witnessed his meticulous restoration of her clocks and knew he would give the Rolls the same careful attention. She first refused to sell but later relented, and he was able to buy it in 1980.

Norman related to me the vehicle's extraordinary history, which I have reviewed with his son, Roger. Despite my research efforts, the following story may be apocryphal.

R. C. Cowan of Oshawa, Ontario had purchased a new 1919 Rolls from the British factory. Later a traffic accident had resulted in extensive front-end damage, which had been repaired at the Rolls Royce factory in Springfield, Massachusetts during the early 1930s. Not all 1919 replacement parts were still available, and some 1930 parts had been adapted to repair the car. The most visible were two new Scintilla lights replacing the original damaged Lucas "King of the Road" headlights.

It had been driven for a few years then left exposed to the elements and deteriorated until its sole function was to support the end of a clothesline in a Dartmouth back yard. For four years the vehicle sat unprotected from the weather and subject to vandalism. The body rusted badly, the engine seized, and instruments were stolen. It was a sad sight when Lieutenant Commander R. A. Creery came upon it in 1947. He approached the owner, who refused to sell him the car, but finally agreed to allow him the use of the vehicle, if he would rebuild the body and engine, making it driveable again.

Despite not having ownership of the car, Creery and two buddies, Steel and Page, decided to do the necessary basic repairs. As a reward, during their 1948 annual summer leave, they would be allowed to tour with the Rolls across North America to British Columbia and back. They worked constantly from September to June. By salvaging parts from any type of vehicle that could be made to function, the Rolls became drivable again. As planned, they took their transcontinent dream trip, an account of which Creery published in the May 1949 copy of the English magazine *The Motorcar*. Reading the account of their trip today, it seems more like an endurance test than a pleasure outing.

Despite having proved itself by the marathon trip, the Rolls was again left exposed to the elements. The owner apparently did not wish to sell or rebuild it but must have tired of potential buyers coming to her door, for when she moved to Annapolis, she hid the Rolls by building her house around it. When purchased by Norman, it had been mostly forgotten. To enable him to take his exciting new treasure home and begin the restoration, part of an enclosing wall of the house had to be removed and repaired.

Authentic replacement parts could only be located on extremely rare, junked Rolls-Royce cars. Norman found one, a 1920 model, in Charlottetown, Prince Edward Island. At one time, this car had belonged to Lord Byng, Governor General of Canada. In 1929, Lockie MacKinnon, an aircraft mechanic and pilot, acquired the car and drove it for three years. On one occasion, while flying, he was forced to make an emergency landing in a field near Ottawa. In order to get airborne again, he used one of the Rolls-Royce "King of the Road" Lucas headlights to mark the end of the field. This "runway light" remained behind in the field, leaving the car with only one headlight.

In 1932, an axle and two wheels were utilized in the construction of an aeroplane trailer. Fortunately, Lockie carefully preserved the engine, steering wheel, instruments, and even the single remaining Lucas headlight—all of which Norman was able to acquire.

Over the next three years, Norman and his son, Roger, made annual sojourns to the giant Antique Automobile Show and Flea Market in Hersey, Pennsylvania, where they found many needed parts, but not the coveted Lucas headlight. During the closing hours of the 1983 show, they came upon a tent selling only headlights, displayed by a Canadian dealer. Among the over two hundred pairs of antique lights was a lonely orphan light, which appeared to be exactly what was needed. Back in his workshop, as Norman removed years of accumulated dirt from his new acquisition, he found serial numbers. Excitedly he searched the original light and found it also had serial numbers. They were identical. Amazingly, during the fifty years they had been separated, no one had discarded either light, and now, unbelievably, the two were together again.

Norman spent many hours returning the car to a like-new condition. He did much of the work himself, even redoing what had been done by professionals if their work had not met his high standards. Once he had the restoration complete, he enjoyed driving and showing his car. At times he would dress in a chauffer's hat and jacket and take couples in his open Rolls to the train station to begin their honeymoons, or high school graduates to their proms.

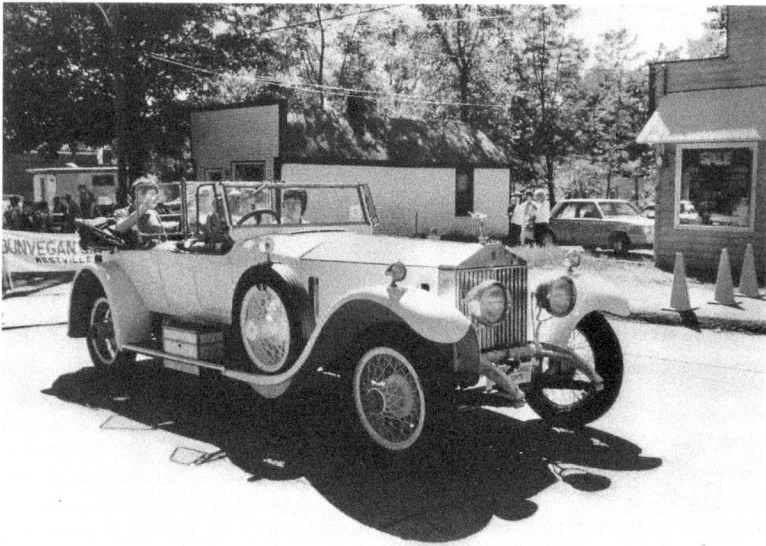

Norman Phinney driving his 1920 Rolls Royce Silver Ghost.
Photo: Oliver Cogswell

The Rolls has since changed hands again and is back home in Britain. I now know the origin of the Rolls-Royce urban legend of my youth. I still do not know the origin of those early dates hand-written inside my clock.

Cars I Have Known

During my pre-teen years I enjoyed accompanying my father on his visits to car dealerships. This was a frequent occurrence for it seemed there was always one of our vehicles that needed replacement. Now that the wartime restriction on the number of civilian automobiles manufactured had been lifted, we could replace the tired old Ford Prefect. Dad and I decided to go to Middleton to examine the expensive Hudson. Leaving our Prefect parked outside, we entered the dealership. None of the salesmen showed any interest in us, until we asked to have the black demonstrator with white wall tires, displayed on the showroom floor, unlocked, so we could sit in it. Our request was refused. We were told the interior had to be kept clean for a potential buyer. Our cheap Prefect, apparently, had indicated to them that Dad, even though dressed in his customary three-piece suit, was not that buyer. "Even a cat can look at a queen," my father commented as we left.

To my amazement when I returned home from school the following day, my clothing soaked through from a heavy rainstorm, there was the black Hudson its whitewalls now coated with mud, parked in front of our house. The salesman was in the office, urging my amused father to take the car for a demonstration drive. He explained to dad that when we were in the showroom, he had not known he was a doctor. My father refused the offer, his excuse being he was afraid his shoes would dirty the interior. I realized, sadly, the Hudson appealed to us, but the dealership did not.

When I began medical school in 1955, my father bought me a 1931 Chev with a cruising speed of thirty-five miles per hour. It had been stored for some time, and after I replaced the wooden driver side doorpost, did an engine valve job, and had it repainted, it served me well. I appreciated the freedom this car provided me.

It allowed me to have my meals at the fraternity, but it did have its problems—especially mechanical brakes, which required frequent adjustment. During the winter I never knew on which wheel the brakes might be frozen, or in what direction the car would be pulled by the brakes still functioning. At times all four wheels were covered with ice, leaving me with no brakes at all. To stop, I would slow the car down then use the engine and the non-synchromesh gears to further slow the car, until I could finally stop the vehicle completely by striking the curb. This worked even on steep Halifax streets. For snow tires, I wrapped old ropes around the wheels and through the spokes. I learned to shift from second to third gears without using the clutch by adjusting the engine speed. I convinced some class-mates the transmission was "semi-automatic." The neighbour across the street was not as pleased with my car as I was; he asked me not to park in front of his house, as he feared his neighbours might think my old car was his.

Alden, a classmate, while hitching a ride in my car, bragged he owned a 1949 Ford which was far newer and nicer than my '31 Chev, but admitted he could not afford to drive it during the university year. He needed his car during each summer break, when he became a door-to-door Fuller Brush salesman. Little did his customers know this Fuller Brushman would soon become their physician. The beginning of our fourth year saw us perfecting our histories and physicals. The ward patients, on whom we practiced, were referred not only from the city but also from all over the province. We were required to examine them, then present our physical findings complete with a diagnosis and a suggested treatment plan.

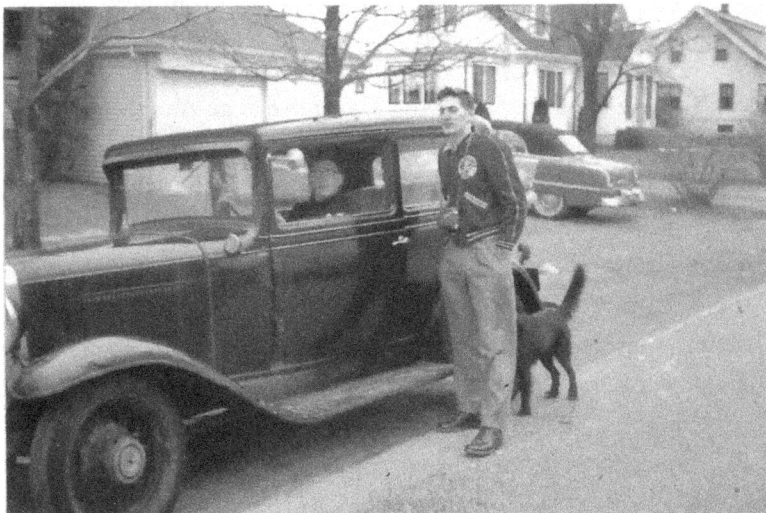

My 1931 Chev. Oliver in the car talking to Eric.
Photo: David Cogswell

Most of our volunteer patients were tired by the time we introduced ourselves. Prior to our visit, they had driven to the city and found the hospital. After an intensive interrogation by the admission clerk, they had been sent to the X-ray department for a mandatory miniature chest film, which was screening for TB. From there, guided by a "Probie" (nurse in training), the patients migrated to the ward where street clothes were exchanged for "Johnnie shirts." Once they were safely in bed, the floor nurse arrived and introduced herself, followed by the head nurse who did the same.

These interviews were often interrupted by the arrival of the medical team, the Head of Service and the Resident physician, each doing cursory exams and explaining coming procedures. The last to visit was the intern who spent an hour doing the formal history and physical. Following all this activity, as fourth year medical students, we were required to practice on these patients. Alden, sent to do his assignment, found his exhausted patient sound asleep and had to shake him awake. The startled man stared at him in disbelief, then exclaimed: "My Gooooddddd!!! . . . The Fuller Brushman!"

One evening in 1963, on impulse, I stopped at an American Motors' dealership to look at a new American Rambler. The only salesman on duty quickly materialized at my side, made an appraisal of my ailing Volkswagen "Bug" and offered me an amazingly good trade offer. The deal was only good for that evening. Reassuring the salesman I would return, I raced home to review this offer with my father. Dad become more and more interested as I recounted the events, then closed his correspondence, and asked where my new car was parked, as he wanted a drive. I explained I had not yet bought the car.

"Then let's go get it," he said, and off we went.

The salesman, pleased to see us, quickly had the contract in order. Backup lights and an outside rear view mirror, front seatbelts, all options were included free of charge. These would be ordered and installed on their arrival. Accepting my personal cheque for the car, he asked us to pay as much in cash as we could, which he needed "to pay the men, as it was the end of the week." We gave him all the cash we had and my cheque for the remainder, left the Volkswagen, and went home in my new car.

I returned a few days later for the installation of my lights and mirror. When the dealership owner saw me, he asked where I had bought the car. Surprised, I answered I had bought it from his dealership. He looked at the car and said, "Yes . . . we had a cream-coloured one like that . . . "

I produced my receipt to confirm my ownership. He studied it with care. Confused, I suggested he confirm things with his salesman.

"Oh . . . he no longer works here . . . but . . . we will honour the terms of the sale."

During the fall of 1968 my negotiations with the local Chrysler dealer to purchase a modest four-door sedan suitable for a country doctor, were quickly complicated. The provincial government announced it was adding a 15 percent sales tax to automobiles, which was to take effect in a few days.

I called the dealership and bought the car.

When I arrived to leave my trade-in, do the paperwork, and take my new car home, I was told it had been sold, as were all the new cars on the lot. I was upset, to console me he said he had a demonstrator on order for himself. As he had the VIN number, this would allow him to sell it to me before the tax came into effect, and because of our misunderstanding he would also give a large discount.

I bought the car, sight unseen.

When it arrived it was a two-door, 1969 Dodge Charger, 440 magnum engine with double noisy exhausts, bright red with a bumblebee stripe around the rear, identical to the muscle car later profiled on the TV series *The Dukes of Hazzard*. I was horrified when I first saw it, but it became my favourite car. It had so much power it could spin its tires at almost any speed, so was able to pull trailers easily, but gave good mileage with my driving, as it needed to be driven cautiously.

They delivered it to my house on a Friday afternoon when we were going to Halifax. An RCMP car followed us in our new car for fifty miles, perhaps expecting us to do our version of *The Dukes of Hazzard*. A warning for me to always drive the Charger carefully.

Privacy & Communication

I have always been intrigued by communications: how they worked, and their relationship to privacy. Society's needs and demands constantly evolved throughout the time my grandfather and father practiced medicine and have continued to change during my lifetime. Dramatic improvements in electronics and means of travel have fuelled major changes in our concept of privacy. The requirements of our forefathers living together in small villages were very different from what we now need in our world village.

The older generations had little concern for privacy as we understand it. Communication was always more important than privacy. During their years in practice neither my father nor my grandfather recognised any need to provide soundproofing between their offices and their waiting areas. My extensive efforts to soundproof my office amused my father. His tiny waiting area contained a built-in bench with a hinged top and two chairs. We children called the bench our "toy box." To get our toys we had to ask the waiting patents to stand. The seating space was so limited that on Saturday nights patient seating extended into our kitchen. In the summer the whole crowded area became unbearably hot, augmented by the wood fire in the kitchen stove, heating water for our baths. There was no privacy for either patients or our family. They knew us, and we knew our father's patients, so it was an all-inclusive family practice.

Our large oak phone was mounted on the waiting room wall. Any calls, either personal or medical, were overheard by the patients.

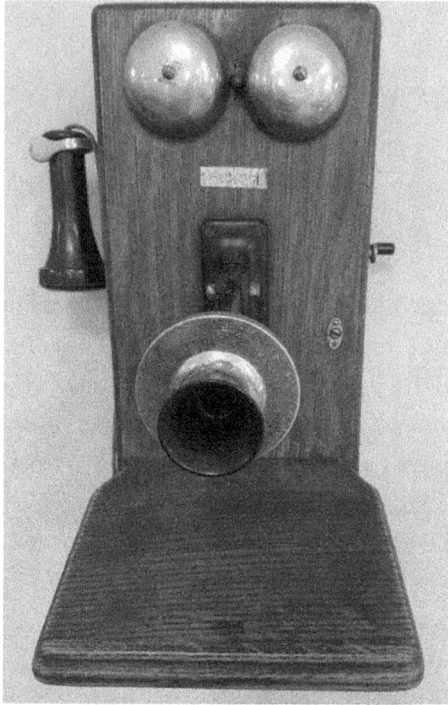

Waiting Room Phone
Cogswell Photo

All telephones at that time were on "party-lines." To use the phone, you listened in to see if the line was busy; if it was, you asked how long the phone would be in use. Usually there was an offer to call you when the line was free. If your call was urgent you were expected to say, "Please hang up. I need to call the doctor." Once your call had time to go through, you frequently heard clicks, as curious neighbours listened in to get the news firsthand. There was no privacy, as anyone on the line had only to lift their receiver to hear the conversation.

My uncle Fred remembered how the sound decreased, making it more and more difficult to communicate, as increasing numbers of people listened in to get the local gossip firsthand. He knew each household, who was wheezing, who had a clock ticking, who was knitting, who had the barking dog, but never did discover whose rocking chair creaked. Grandfather had two phones and two numbers, as his home was located where two different party lines met.

At our home, "the doctor's house," we were lucky because the only other person on our line was Grandmother Cogswell. To call her, you turned the crank for a long and a short ring, our ring was a long and two shorts. Before we left for a visit to the Killam grandparents, Dad would push a button and turn the crank to get the operator. "I will be at Kay's father's, if anyone needs me." The operator knew his voice, knew who Kay's father was, and the number. She doubled as a telephone answering service and always got a large box of chocolates for Christmas.

Although offering little privacy, these party lines helped circulate community news and could be helpful when physicians were forced to make home calls in stormy weather. When school was cancelled by a storm, I often saw the drama unfold. Dad would be called to the phone. Someone was desperately sick. Voices of many:

"Can the doctor come?"

"What are the roads like, can I get there?"

Neighbours from all along the route would offer advice:

"No one has got up the Harbourville Mountain, don't try it!"

"As you know I live on the Black Rock Mountain. The plow hasn't been up yet, but earlier someone got up with a truck. They are shovelling two stuck cars, but I think you will be able to get around them if you are careful."

"I think you can make it."

"I will have the guys here, so when you see him go by, call me, and we will go down in the hollow where the snow is drifting and push him through."

"Tell him not to stop."

I had to beg a bit to go on these trips, but they were an exciting change from school. Everyone knew Dad kept a car with steel chains over snow tires, ready for these winter trips. The party line was used again to get us through the drifts on our way home.

My grandfather Killam did not have the luxury of this party line help during his early years of practice. He went by horse and sleigh. To prevent the sleigh from getting mired in large snowdrifts he would jump from his seat and heave up on the handrail, lifting the sleigh to make it easier for the horse. He was so strong that on one occasion he pulled the whole rail off the sleigh.

Communications were slower in my grandfather's day. He spent a great deal of his time traveling by horse and buggy, or by sleigh, to various homes where his services were required. Commercial radio was not available until the mid-20s, and the nearest library was in distant Wolfville. His highly prized 1913 *Encyclopaedia Britannica* and newspapers were his only contact with the outside world. For assistance in dealing with difficult, complicated illnesses, he corresponded directly with consultants by mail.

On Saturdays and on Sundays after church, the field next to grandfather's house was full of wagons. The men tended the horses and gossiped while wives and children awaited their turn in the waiting room. The families knew each other and shared their medical and other problems. They supported and helped each other. My grandfather, who knew their most intimate secrets, must have felt a moral duty to protect his patients. I was told by one of his former patients, later one of mine, that the whole community watched my grandfather running after a wagon while the owner whipped up the horses to get away. The bystanders knew and approved that my grandfather was trying to accost the man in retribution for wife abuse.

When I began my practice, telephone service had greatly improved, and I was able to get a private line, even though only party lines were available to most customers. During the first year of practice, I had an extension, a sort of party line, put into my great-aunt Lena's house, and she became my telephone answering service, something not available at that time. Each village had its own telephone exchange and operator. Long distance charges were levied when an operator was needed to go from one exchange to another.

Shortly after I began practice, Doctor Paul Kinsman and I established the first call system in the valley, by alternating weekend and evening calls. We had telephone extensions installed in each other's home offices, allowing our receptionists to answer both office lines directly when on call. This released Aunt Lena from her answering service. We took our own hospital, late evening, and night calls, even when technically not on call. Our innovative telephone company hardware, plus the many long-distance charges, were expensive. Even a call to the hospital, six miles away, was long distance, as were calls to Greenwood. My voice became familiar, and I was on a first name basis with many operators who recognized any strange voice that might try to bill a long-distance call to me by pretending to be me. If it was not my voice, they would offer to call the customer back once the connection was made. Immediately the callers would ask them to cancel the call.

Even with our efforts to have good communications there was always the human factor. Paul became elected as the local Member of the Legislative Assembly, and his housekeeper referred his night calls to me while he was in Halifax. He returned and ran his office on weekends.

One Wednesday I met the housekeeper going to the post office. "I am so mad!" she said.

"What happened?" I asked.

"Last night the phone woke me at three a.m.," she said. "The caller asked if Dr. Kinsman was there. I explained he was in Halifax attending the sitting of the legislature, and Dr. Cogswell is on call. There was a long pause before the voice asked, 'When will he be back?' I told him, 'Not until Friday evening, but Dr. Cogswell is on call.'" There was another long pause, she explained, before his response: "Then I guess it can wait."

My fascination for wireless communication began when I was quite young. I was introduced to a radio "shack" for the first time while visiting my friend Billy. There I saw his father, earphones clamped tightly to his ears, speaking enthusiastically into a microphone and clicking on a key. There were racks in the room full of glowing tubes, switches, and cooling fans. He was a radio "ham." I soon found my uncle Fred was one as well. My uncle and I spent many interesting evenings together while he explained how his homemade equipment sent messages over radio waves around the world. I, of course, wanted to become a ham as well. I got a key and learned Morse code, earning a Cub badge. I soon realized it would not be possible for me to become a ham for some years due to the cost, the need for equipment, space, and the inherent dangers of the electrical equipment to my younger siblings. It was not until March 2002 that I earned my ham call letters which are VE1 ETC and VA1 DC.

Early in my medical practice I would return from a home visit only to find another request for a call in the area I had just left. If only I could have been contacted while there. This need led me to explore the possibility of having Citizen Band radio communications. By 1965, Paul Kinsman and I had citizen band transmitters in our homes, cars, and at the hospital switchboard. We obtained "crystals" from the Department of Transport, allowing us the privacy of having our own frequency. This not only improved our efficiency but made house calls and trips to the hospital at night—or in bad weather—safer. We were now available for emergencies from the hospital or the office.

This car radio nearly cost me a patient. I had just completed a call in Greenwood and was leaving for home when my wife Heide reached me with a request for a house call. The timing was perfect because I was almost in front of the home in question. When I went to the door, the woman took one look at me and said, "I no longer want you to be my doctor . . . you drive too fast."

A Family Vacation (or, How to Smuggle Children)

In the spring of 1972, I received notice that the College of Family Physicians of Canada and the General Practitioners of the UK had planned a joint annual meeting in London, England. Since Heide's parents were going to Mallorca for the winter that year, we realized we would be able to combine the two events. No one family would be responsible for entertaining, as occurred when we visited Heide's family back home in Germany, or they visited us in Canada. Each family would be independent, and with everyone on vacation we would have more free time for each other. It would be a great opportunity to have a relaxing visit. I could even claim part of my trip as a business expense by remaining in London for the conference. It had been a stressful year. We welcomed and looked forward to having time together as a family, with no cares for the next two weeks.

My mother drove us to the airport late in the evening for our overnight flight to Europe. As it was already late, she left immediately to return home. We held tickets to Heathrow with a connecting flight to Mallorca, where Heide's parents would be waiting to meet us.

Our euphoria quickly metamorphosed to anxiety when the Air Canada ticket agent checked our passports. "Where is the passport for the little boy?" she asked.

I thought back; we had gone to Barbados with our son when he was six weeks old. "He must be on my wife's passport," I answered.

The agent looked on Heide's passport and Eric's name was not there. Suddenly I remembered that we had taken him to Barbados without a passport. The travel agent had informed us our child would be exempt for that trip, there would not be enough time between his birth and when we were leaving to obtain a passport. We had traveled so little and were so naïve. Obviously, we should have had a passport. Luckily the customs agents both going into Barbados and coming back to Canada were good-natured and kind. They realized we were tourists, and Heide was a nursing mother. With warnings to have him added to Heide's passport on our return, they allowed us to have our planned vacation. Now he was two-and-a-half, and our failure to acquire a passport for him would cause us major grief.

We did not want to cancel our trip. Heide and I had no way of contacting her parents who would be meeting us in Mallorca. They would be very upset if no one came. I told her to go ahead with our two girls, and I would take Eric and return to Halifax, where I would obtain a passport. We would follow them the next day. Unhappy but seeing no alternative, we separated. Heide took Sonya and Karen and boarded the plane. With a sinking heart, I stayed behind with Eric.

I had spoken earlier to a customs agent at the airport who warned me if I went on the plane without a passport for Eric, we would both be sent back as soon as the plane landed in London. I spoke to them again, to learn there was no passport office and no way to quickly get a passport in Halifax. I then went to the Air Canada ticket agent to obtain tickets for the next flight to London. There were no flights the next day, nor any flights for several days. With the difficulty and high cost of flights, they suggested I take the risk and go with my family. The plane was held, the ramp replaced, and I ran with my luggage under one arm, and my son nestled under the other. We were very happy to be reunited as a family; but what was to happen to us?

I did not sleep on the overnight trip. By now all the passengers knew of our predicament and we received a great deal of conflicting advice. The steward even suggested a bribe might work. He advised me not to try to bribe the English customs officials, but we might be able to bribe the Spanish. I had no intentions of doing either. The children slept. We did not. We looked through all the papers we had with us. We had no evidence of his being our child. Despite the fact I was a doctor and had all the forms in my office, I had not even added him to my Medicare card. To my horror, we had no proof of little Eric being part of our family.

With all the anxiety and all the suggestions, the trip seemed shorter than usual. We landed in Heathrow, where first we expected to go through English and then through Spanish customs. I saw a sign that said, "Passengers in Transit to Europe." To my great relief, our tickets were all that were required to get us on the plane for the last leg of our journey. We walked past the line waiting for the British customs officials. One barrier less, I thought.

Once we were safely landed in Mallorca, at the entrance to the customs area I saw only one agent sitting in what resembled a phone booth, in the open hall. I collected the passports and told eleven-year-old Sonya, the eldest, to take Eric's hand and walk through into Spain, to her waiting grandparents. I spoke to the official to distract him while he examined our passports. He did not notice there were only four passports for five people. We were in Spain.

The visit was wonderful despite the cool spring weather. We had been hoping for warmer weather but spending time visiting the grandparents and the cosmopolitan crowd made the trip memorable. We had interesting experiences juggling different languages. On one occasion, my father-in-law, Vati, decided he needed some cough medicine. Although he could manage in German, Low German, Afrikaans, Dutch and Latin, he did not know Spanish or English. He took me with him to the pharmacist since I spoke English and understood the components of the medications. The pharmacist could speak very little of any of the languages we could provide. In frustration, Vati exclaimed in German, "What languages can you speak?" The pharmacist's reply, in English, was, "I speak perfect Spanish."

I never dared leave little Eric's side during the vacation. It was frightening to realize he could wander off, and I would have a difficult time finding him, not knowing the country or the language. With no passport and no identification, how could I identify him if he was lost? How could I prove he was mine if he was found? I did not even have his picture. He became "Daddy's boy," and we both enjoyed it. Our return trip was booked with an overnight stay in London. I tried desperately to get the flights for Heide and the girls booked straight through to Canada, like our arrival itinerary, and avoid the UK. Nothing was available. We would all have to stay overnight in London and go through English customs twice. We needed some evidence Eric was ours. I called Ethel Whitman, who was a surrogate mother to our family. She was also coming to London for the conference with her employer, Dr. Paul Kinsman. I asked her to bring a picture of our family with Eric, or at least some evidence he was ours. She said she had a family picture and would try to get a birth certificate. She called me back to tell me she had no success getting the birth certificate but would bring the picture. I asked her to leave it at the BOAC desk at the airport, so that on our arrival in London I would have it to prove Eric was our child. Hopefully this would get us through English customs.

Suddenly, sadly, the vacation was over. We had to leave the grandparents and Mallorca; I had to go to the conference, Heide and the children had to return to Canada. The spectre of two trips through English customs still hung over us. We all had to spend the night in London, and the next day my family would take the morning flight to Canada.

At the Mallorca airport, I saw the single customs agent in the same confined space as when we arrived. Sonya again took Eric by the hand and walked past the custom agent. A little distraction by me, four passports, and all five of us were out of Spain and soon landed in London.

Now for the careful, incorruptible, imperturbable British custom agents. I went to the BOAC desk and asked if there was an envelope there for me. "We are an airline not a travel agency, sir," I was told. "Any envelope or personal message is probably on the message pillar." The pillar she indicated was just beyond the customs desk. Sonya, who seemed by now to be enjoying her part in our deceptions, took Eric by the hand and past the bored agent, who checked the four passports. Lucky for us, he too did not notice there were five of us. I found the envelope containing our pictures on the message pillar. We were in London.

We arrived quite early at our hotel. Although it was raining, we went on an exciting walking tour past the parliament buildings and admired the area.

The next day was going to be difficult for Heide. She had only three passports for four people. The youngest one, Eric, was expecting to be carried on board by his father. I went with them to the airport to see them safely on the plane. Hoping to prevent any attention-getting tears, I carried Eric and accompanied them as far as was permitted. When it was their turn to go through customs, I said to Eric—whose toilet training was fresh in his mind—"I have to go to the washroom. You take Sonya's hand." And then I left without any fuss or goodbyes. Heide used our time-tested border techniques, customs did not notice one passport was missing, and all was well. She relaxed. The deception had worked. She was in the departure lounge, and the only hurdle left was the customs officials in Halifax.

But as they were boarding the plane, the Air Canada stewardess asked to see Eric's passport. Heide replied, "We goofed. I do not have one, but I have a family picture." The only response was, "You sure did!"

On their return entry to Canada, the customs agents again did not notice there were only three passports for four passengers, and they were safely home.

I remained in London and enjoyed attending the lectures which began early in the morning and continued late into the evening. Dr. Kinsman and I attended most together.

Eager to see my family, I arrived early at the airport for my return trip. The Air Canada ticket agent asked for my smallpox vaccination certificate. I told her I did not need one, as smallpox had been eliminated from the world. I knew because I was a doctor and there was no longer a requirement for a certificate. She told me a smallpox outbreak had occurred following a lab accident, and yes, I required a certificate to re-enter Canada. I was sent to health control to be re-vaccinated and receive my certificate.

Having removed my shirt as ordered by the nurse, I offered my left deltoid to the physician, waiting with the needle. He held my arm, looked at me, and said, "Where are you from?"

"Canada."

"Where in Canada?"

"Nova Scotia."

"Where in Nova Scotia?"

"The Annapolis Valley".

"You are Dr. Cogswell, aren't you?"

Astonished, I looked at him and realised he had interviewed me in Aylesford the previous year, as he had wished at that time to immigrate to Nova Scotia. I had encouraged him to come since we needed more physicians. He told me he had developed health issues which made him unable to do a country practice, and he had subsequently joined the British Health Service. I got a free vaccination.

I went to buy my duty-free liquor. In those days you did not get your purchase until you were seated in the plane. As names were called you identified yourself and were presented with your duty-free goods. When I boarded the plane, I was given an aisle seat next to a woman whose husband had the window seat. We had just begun a polite conversation, when abruptly "Dr. Cogswell" was called. I identified myself.

The woman next to me looked at me in disbelief.

"I didn't believe there was a Dr. Cogswell. You really are Dr. Cogswell? I am so happy there is a Dr. Cogswell. You really are Dr. Cogswell? I am so relieved!"

Quite surprised and taken aback, I asked for an explanation. When she and her husband had arrived in London for the same medical conference, a small bald man (Dr. Kinsman) had approached and asked if she was going to the terminal where planes arrived from the continent. She said they were. He then passed her an envelope and asked her to post it on a bulletin board, on her arrival at that terminal. It was important, for it contained a picture needed to help Dr. Cogswell get a child into London. This would save the man from making the trip to the other terminal.

"I took the picture to the other terminal and put it on the bulletin post as he requested," she said. "Later I read in the paper about a crime ring, smuggling children into England, and was afraid I'd gotten involved."

Now her conscience was clear, I had my duty-free liquor, and we were all heading, unhindered, towards home.

Daughter Suzanne

As we left the courtroom of the Appeals Division of the Supreme Court of Nova Scotia in the fall of 1984, it seemed our ordeal was over. Our lawyer had won our "test case" with the Municipality of Kings County, even though a legal team from the Province of Nova Scotia had joined the prosecution against us. They had tried to prove that we, Heide, and I, were the ones who required welfare—not our nineteen-year-old daughter, Suzanne, who was born a microcephalic. The municipality, in their efforts to force us to be financially responsible for our adult child's institutional care, had taken us through the Nova Scotia court system, and they had lost. My father had always urged us to negotiate solutions to problems and avoid going to court, but this time my efforts at negotiation had failed. I now understood how fortunate we were in Canada to have universal basic rights and a legal system that was able to support them. We had won not only for ourselves but for all other Nova Scotian parents, both past and future, who had severely disabled adult children.

Although Suzanne had a small head at birth, the severity of her disability only became obvious as she began missing her developmental milestones. She never learned to speak. To try and discover the cause of her problem, we had her and ourselves accessed by a variety of pediatricians, virologist, geneticists. They did not find any cause for her abnormality; it was a spontaneous sporadic event which would not recur in other pregnancies or in our descendants.

Suzanne required twenty-four-hour care and observation. This became more difficult for us to provide as she grew older and became more mobile. She loved music and put her head on the piano while it was being played. She knew food was prepared on the stove, and, when hungry, might try to put her hand on the elements. She could open the door and go outside, but did not know how to come back inside, even though she was cold. She would wander at night when we were sleeping. The pediatricians advised we place her in a children's home for her safety. Seeing no alternative, we were assessed by a social worker who agreed Suzanne needed to be in a home for the disabled, and explained that the province paid for her care. All children in Nova Scotia were required to go to school, and she would be taught basic things, such as dressing and feeding herself. We admitted her to the Digby Children's Home (DCH) and paid the same monthly fee toward her care as all the other parents. We frequently visited her there and had her home on holidays.

When she was a few months short of seventeen years of age, the administrator of the DCH interviewed us, and informed us that when Suzanne reached seventeen, she would be considered an adult and could no longer remain in a children's home. She would have to be moved to a home for disabled adults. We needed to arrange with Social Services for her placement. I asked if she could be an exception and be allowed to stay in her present home, where she was content. Suzanne was very small and most likely would not grow any larger; she appeared the same size as the children around her. We were concerned that she might not be able to adapt to a new situation with much larger adults. The administrator told us he was not permitted to do placements; these were the responsibility of the municipality from which the individual came. Suzanne could only be placed in a home for disabled adults by Kings County Social Services.

Unfortunately, I was not on good terms with the director of this department. We had previously clashed over his placements, one of which was a man sent to a small rural nursing home where I served as the doctor. The staff called me to see the new admission, who seemed depressed. I found a dejected, unilingual, French-speaking Acadian man, away from friends and family, sitting isolated in an English-speaking environment, unable to communicate with anyone around him. I became exasperated, and at one point accused the Director of being more concerned about his budget than his clients. I managed, with great difficulty, to get the patient placed in a more appropriate location.

Following our application to have Suzanne placed in an adult home, a Social Services worker called and made an appointment to interview us in our home, not in the municipal office. I wondered why. Perhaps the Director had forgiven me and was helping me place my daughter, in consideration for all my years working for the municipality, as the on-call doctor for their new 250 bed Kings County Hospital (KCH) in Waterville, now the Kings Regional Rehabilitation Center. Maybe the Director and the municipal council recognized my contribution in the rehabilitation of the chronically ill patients housed in the KCH, who were previously seen as untreatable. These were the people I had feared in my childhood years, as I watched them walking in circles within their fenced-in prison, while I waited for my father to make his medical visits. Now I, as the Kings County Municipal Hospital KCH physician, was part of the medical, occupational, nursing, and community teams who had been able to treat and discharge about four hundred of these patients back to their home communities over an eight-year period, using new major tranquilizers, more active psychiatric treatment, socialization within the community and the hospital, and hope. In January 1971, MacLean's Magazine claimed the "Kings County Hospital has been transformed from a dead-end mental institution to one of the nation's most progressive municipal psychiatric treatment centers."

I was soon to learn this home visit was not a reward for my services. When the worker from Social Services arrived, she told us the Director had decided to place Suzanne himself. However, there were some preliminary routine forms that needed to be signed before Suzanne could be considered for admission to any facility for mentally disabled adults. These forms would confirm we agreed to support her indefinitely, as would our estate after our death. They believed my father and I were millionaires, as we were both doctors, and expected me to support my adult daughter. They were certain there would be no problem supporting Suzanne from my earnings, which they would confiscate and use for her support. We would be given a living wage; they would decide the amount. These forms would also give Social Services permission to access our income tax records forever into the future and five years into the past. We were required to provide records of all our debts, savings, investments, and to have our home, cottage, and cars evaluated. If I refused to sign, they would not place my daughter and she would have to leave the children's home. This was the law, others had already signed, and I would have to sign as well.

I asked for copies of the law in question, and to my surprise they were sent to me. I found the municipality was using two unrelated laws. One law stated disabled children in N S were supported financially by the province, with all parents contributing the same nominal amount. When children became seventeen years old, the age of consent in Nova Scotia at that time, they were considered adults, and no longer qualified for this child benefit. The second law stated that an adult with a mental handicap was a child and therefore the parents' responsibility. Social Services had decided to combine the two unrelated laws, in effect making my application for her admission to a home the same as if I was applying for myself. I was not welcome to attend council meetings to defend myself, so I made appointments to speak to two councillors at their homes and was told, "You have lots of money. Now you will just have to live like the rest of us."

Once Suzanne became seventeen years old, I began receiving bills from DCH for her care and requests she be moved to an adult home.

A large community meeting held in Aylesford, and reported on October 6ᵗʰ, 1984, in *The Examiner*, Middleton's newspaper, stated:

> . . . concerns were voiced that Kings County Director of Social Services [. . .] is adamant that Dr. David Cogswell pay the full upkeep for his severely mentally retarded daughter, Suzanne, who is now in a Digby home.
>
> The maximum weekly rate charged under the Social Services Act in Kings County is $25 per week.
>
> The director of Social Services maintains the charge could be as high as $30,000 per year minus Suzanne's disability pension for the rest of Dr. Cogswell's lifetime . . . it was suggested [. . .] was making an example of Dr. Cogswell, to the point of an act of the Social Services which had never in the history of the Social Services been implanted against the parents of retarded children, had been used in the case of Suzanne.

We were summoned to a formal hearing before municipal and provincial welfare officials. I again refused to sign, and they refused to place her. I arranged a meeting with the provincial minister of welfare, who told us he supported his five children, and we should support our child, but he did agree to have Suzanne transferred to an adult home.

It now was obvious that our only hope of having a normal family life was to leave Nova Scotia. My wife Heide had an aunt and three first cousins in Ontario where my brother, his family, my aunt, uncle, and cousins all lived as well. No such draconian laws existed in that province. I obtained my Ontario medical licence. We visited and found very nice home willing to accept Suzanne. She would be eligible for provincial support once she had been an Ontario resident for one year.

Without warning we received a summons; the municipality of Kings County, Nova Scotia sued us for her support. We had to remain in Nova Scotia and protect ourselves in court. If we lost, we would be forced to cover her maintenance, and that ruling might force us to continue her support, even if we moved to another province. I approached a local lawyer who agreed to defend us but volunteered that he expected we would lose. I wanted a defence team that thought we would win. On the advice of a legal friend, I made a scrapbook of the newspaper accounts of our journey to that time and added written comments about each one. We then made an appointment with Mr. Goodfellow, the lawyer our legal friend suggested. Mr. Goodfellow appeared surprised to see a couple enter his office. As a family law specialist, most of his clients were individuals seeking legal advice during divorce hearings. After reviewing my scrap book, he agreed to represent us. Then went on to inform us this was a "test case" which would require extra research and then quoted us his fee.

We were pleased he would represent us and replied we would not hold him to his quote. He could bill us if extra time was required to prepare our defence. The county was determined to win and appealed to the next court level after each loss. Mr. Goodfellow, as he had done the first time, quoted us his fee for our defence, and refused to bill more than his quote. He certainly lived up to his name, being very kind and knowledgeable. I will always be grateful to him for his hard work on our behalf.

I wrote the provincial Association for Mental Retardation, asking for moral support and was disappointed not to receive any reply. A similar letter to the Medical Society revealed they considered this to be my problem, not a medical society problem, and they refused to be involved. I was surprised the only judge to rule against me came from the same community and was a few years ahead of me in school.

Despite these setbacks it was wonderful how much support I received from family, friends, and the community. My brother Eric and friend Dr. Henshaw offered financial help; fortunately, I managed on my own. Dr. Jim Millar went on a talk show in my support. Noreen Clem organized the community meeting with Dr. Henshaw in the chair. A previous patient attending Dalhousie University was taking a class in law where the professor used our case for teaching, I was informed of the class discussions in which students presented possible arguments both for and against my case. A member of the municipal council, who I did not know, was so upset with what the council was doing, that he called me following the in-camera sessions to keep me informed.

Aylesford may lose family physician

by Jackie Fitton

Aylesford may lose its family doctor, Western Kings Memorial hospital may lose its anesthetist if the stubborness by Kings County Social Services and Kings County Council persists, it was said by villagers at the general meeting of Aylesford villagers, held in the fire hall last week.

Concerns were voiced that Kings County director of Social Services, Henry Bourgeois is adamant that Dr. David Cogswell pay the full upkeep for his severely mentally retarded daughter, Suzanne, who is now in a Digby nursing home.

The maximum weekly rate charged under the Social Services Act in Kings County is $25 per week.

The director of Social Services maintains the charge to Dr. Cogswell could be as high as $30,000 per year minus Suzanne's disability pension for the rest of Dr. Cogswell's lifetime. Up to now the province has funded Suzanne. It is Suzanne that is applying, she will be 19 years old October 27 and by law Suzanne is an adult Dr. and Mrs. Cogswell

are applying on behalf of Suzanne, who has no assets of her own, other than a disability pension.

Suzanne by law can obtain a driving licence, drink alcohol and east her vote, in fact she is an adult in the eyes of the law and is of legal

age - but she is an adult only by age and Dr. J.D.A. Henshaw.

Feelings at the general meeting rose when it was suggested Mr. Bourgeois was making an example of point of an act of the social services which

had never in the history of the Social Services been implanted against the parents of retarded children, had been used in the case of Suzanne Kings County council must place. Suzanne

See Aylesford Page 4

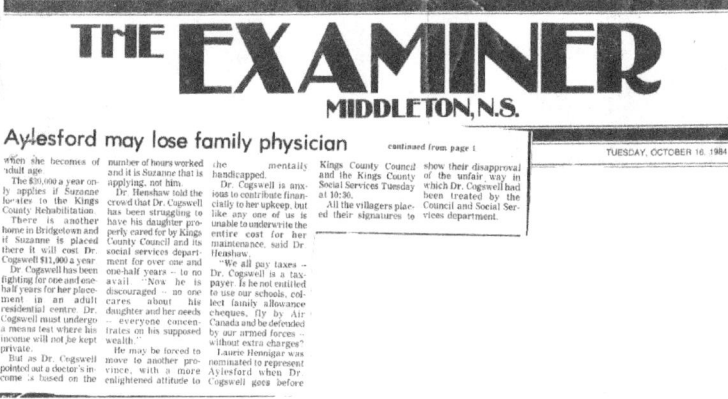

THE EXAMINER
MIDDLETON, N.S.

Aylesford may lose family physician

continued from page 1

when she becomes of adult age.

The $30,000 a year only applies if Suzanne l99ries to the Kings County Rehabilitation.

There is another home in Bridgetown and if Suzanne is placed there it will cost Dr. Cogswell $11,000 a year.

Dr. Cogswell has been fighting for one and one half years for her placement in an adult residential centre. Dr. Cogswell must undergo a means test where his income will not be kept private.

But as Dr. Cogswell pointed out a doctor's income is based on the

number of hours worked and it is Suzanne that is applying, not him.

Dr. Henshaw told the crowd that Dr. Cogswell has been struggling to have his daughter properly cared for by Kings County Council and its social services department.

"We all pay taxes - one-half years - to no avail. "Now he is discouraged - no one cares about his daughter and her needs - everyone concentrates on his supposed wealth."

He may be forced to move to another province, with a more enlightened attitude to Dr. Cogswell goes before

the mentally handicapped.

Dr. Cogswell is anxious to her upkeep. But like any one of us is unable to underwrite the entire cost for her maintenance, said Dr. Henshaw.

"We all pay taxes - Dr. Cogswell is a taxpayer. Is he not entitled to use our schools, collect family allowance cheques, fly by Air Canada and be defended by our armed forces - without extra charges?"

Laurie Hennigar was nominated to represent Aylesford when Dr. Cogswell goes before

Kings County Council and the Kings County Social Services Tuesday at 10:30.

All the villagers have ed their signatures to

show their disapproval of the unfair way in which Dr. Cogswell has been treated by the Council and Social Services department.

TUESDAY, OCTOBER 16, 1984

Newspaper clipping — community support of Dr. David Cogswell.

I learned I had many friends and supporters, and that we all are fortunate to have courts and a legal system that are independent of political pressures. This counterbalance protects us, and allows us all win.

13 Confinements

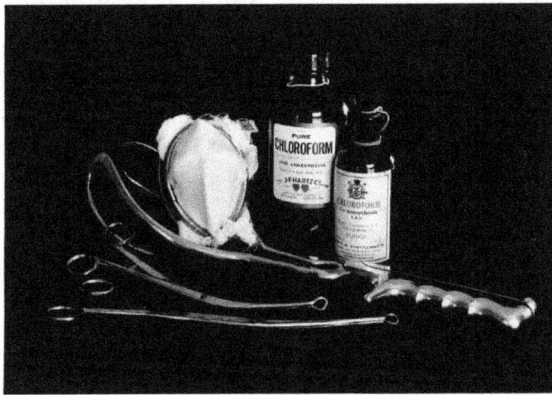

Partial contents of Dr. Laverne's Obestrical Bag

Both my father and grandfather spent a large part of their practice managing "confinements", a general term to describe home deliveries and complications of pregnancies, the term we children frequently heard to explain our father's absence. Prior to the construction of the WKMH, and even after, home births were the norm, mostly for economic reasons. I now wish I had asked my grandfather how he managed—both medically and emotionally—this wonderful but difficult part of his practice. A stroll through any of our cemeteries today reveals that many young women died in childbirth. Sadly, surgical interventions that are now routine had not been available to them.

Both my grandfather and my father carried chloroform, ether, forceps, drugs, and other instruments in their obstetrical and medical bags, but alone, without any trained assistants and such limited equipment, how did they manage those kitchen table emergencies that must have occurred? Home births with slower emergency response times remained the standard during most of my grandfather's and much of my father's working years. Following the construction of our community hospital, routine surgeries were planned, and on-call lists allowed the surgeon, assistant, anaesthesiologists, and the nursing team to be quickly available for obstetrical and other emergencies.

By the time I began my practice the public were taking emergencies directly to the hospital, where nursing and medical care were immediately available, instead of to doctor's offices. Patients who formally said they were treated in "Dr. XYZ's office" now said they were treated "at XYZ hospital," implying the best care came from the latter. Our local surgeon was accosted by parents wanting to know why their child had been taken past a larger hospital, to be treated by him in our smaller one. His reply was, "Madam, patients are referred to physicians, not institutions."

This developing community perception that hospitals treated emergencies hit me one holiday season following a fairy-tale Christmas Eve. All day, warmed by the fireplace and surrounded by presents, we had added ornaments to the tree while snow fell outside. Knowing Santa had filled all the stockings, we went late to bed. The dreaded phone woke me. A patient in labour had arrived at the hospital, and I was to come immediately. I asked why I was needed so early in her labour and was told to look out the window, where I saw the highway and my driveway completely blocked by drifting snow. Knowing the Department of Highway snowplows had managed to transport my patient from her home to the hospital, I called and thanked them, and asked if they would please come for me as well, to do the delivery.

They told me, "Sir, we plow public highways, not private driveways. It is your responsibility to have your yard plowed."

Bewildered, I called the owner of the local service station and asked if he could get me to the hospital. He said his Jeep would be unable to go even one car length in the deep snow. In desperation, I called Ronald Baltzer, the nearby farm equipment dealer, to see if he would take me, with his big tractor.

"It's Christmas," he said.

"My Christmas too," I answered.

"Walk down to the highway and as soon as I get my big tractor running, I will pick you up."

Despite the fact there were two cars marooned in the snow in front of his home (with the owners asleep in his living room), he came, took me to the hospital, and then continued taking staff to and from the hospital to their homes. We were fortunate to have excellent nurses, one of whom had delivered the patient prior to my arrival. I had three deliveries that Christmas day.

There was a large indigent component to my father's practice. He would not refuse anyone just because they could not pay. This policy and his excellent obstetrical reputation resulted in a caseload of up to three hundred deliveries a year. How he managed this I do not understand, but he must have been chronically sleep-deprived. Few pregnant women at that time made prenatal visits. Frequently, the first realization he was caring for a pregnant patient was a call from the hospital, or more commonly from a home, informing him he was urgently needed for the delivery.

Many of the homes he visited had a lower level of cleanliness than that found in a hospital setting. Some mornings, as we were leaving for school, Mother would be tearing the marital bed apart saying, "There he is . . . I got him!" And "Fleas don't bite your father; he just brings them home to bite me."

Dad once told me how he attended a delivery in a house so cluttered he did not dare sit until he found a relatively clean hardwood chair. The woman's labour progressed slowly, and with night coming on, he was offered a couch on which to rest. He politely refused, his excuse being he needed to stay in the chair to properly follow the labour. Even sitting up he began to doze, gradually feeling his arms and legs going to sleep, but the rest of his body was unable to follow, as each time he nodded off, the movement of his head jolted him wide awake. Finally, with dawn breaking, Dad was offered breakfast. Looking at the piles of unwashed dishes, he said his usual breakfast was just black coffee.

On another occasion, while monitoring another labour, not only did his arms and legs go to sleep, but he also went to sleep as well. This time a baby's cry woke him. When questioned why they had not wakened him to attend to the delivery, they replied that everything seemed to be going well, and he had appeared so tired, they decided he needed the sleep more than they needed his help for the delivery.

It was so unusual for my father to be away from home that I still remember the trip he made for a delivery "over the mountain," from which he did not return for several days. Leaving home during a snowstorm he utilized his legendary driving skills manoeuvring the "winter car" with chains up the "Harbourville Mountain," around the steep U-turn known to locals as the "ox-bow," past cars mired in the drifts of snow, to the top of the mountain. From there it was downhill to Harbourville (on the Bay of Fundy) where Mable Spicer, a former nurse, operated a hotel, restaurant, general store, and post office. It was the hub of the village. Shortly after his arrival, the roads became impassable. He realized he was "storm stayed," not only with the woman in labour, but with several other pregnant women who had come to Spicers as well. They wanted to be near the doctor in case they began their labour, not marooned at home. The summer holiday hotel had become a maternity hospital.

Harbourville remained snowed in for days. Prior to the opening of the road, two men driving a team of horses broke through the drifts to bring Dad home. They planned to return with badly needed supplies. Excitedly we saw the procession come up the town's main street to our front yard, Dad with his medical bags sitting on a child's bobsled behind the two horses, men with shovels walking alongside. We children secretly envied Dad this trip. Our only chance for a similar ride behind a horse was to beg Aubrey to let us sit next to him on the simple wooden plow he used to clear the town sidewalks. The "winter car" remained in Harbourville "until spring," my mother used to say, but most likely for one or two weeks.

I was concerned there might be confusion having two Dr. Cogswells if I opened an office near my father. Far more worrisome was the lack of specialist backup so easily available to my classmates who were practicing in the city. To avoid confusion with our two names, the nursing director immediately gave me the nickname "Dr. David." My two years extra training gave me some confidence in both surgery and internal medicine, but there were no full-time obstetricians or anaesthetists within the valley. I needed to expand my obstetrical and anaesthetic competence to make my family practice as comprehensive, useful, and satisfying as that of my father and grandfather. My father was considered the most proficient local practitioner in both of these areas and his willingness to mentor me provided the necessary security. For some time, I also spent my Friday mornings unofficially in Halifax operating theatres, being mentored by kind anaesthesiologists.

I opened my practice in Aylesford, a village midway between Greenwood, the military base, and Berwick, where both the hospital and my father's practice were located. Being near military families who were younger and who were posted here from outside areas allowed me to quickly establish a practice.

Entering the hospital for a delivery one night, I was met by the supervisor, who told me the labour was progressing well, but slowly. There would be enough time, prior to my seeing the patient, for me to visit the admission clerk, who urgently wanted to speak to me. Intrigued, I went to her desk to learn that despite being in labour, my patient on arrival had been evasive when asked to provide her doctor's name.

"Well, I'm not sure," she said.

"You surely must have had a doctor for your prenatal care?"

"Yes, but I am not sure I trust Dr. Cogswell anymore. I just called to let him know I was having contractions and to see what I should do. He was awfully vague. After I was speaking to him awhile, he said 'I think you're pregnant.' Can you believe it? I had been seeing him every month. I thought he must have been half asleep and kept on talking to get him awake. Suddenly Dr. Cogswell said, 'I think you're in labour; you should go to the hospital.' He didn't remember I was pregnant or even who I was! He didn't even sound like the same man! Is there something wrong with Dr. Cogswell? Does he drink?"

At that time there were three separate telephone exchanges in Kingston, Aylesford, and Berwick providing telephone coverage over the fifteen-kilometre distance from the Greenwood Military Base to the hospital. The expectant mother in question had inadvertently called the Berwick exchange and spoken to my father, thinking it was me. Both the admission clerk and the supervisor had tried to explain the problem to the patient, but she remained unconvinced. She was concerned the staff had invented the story to protect me.

Working with one's father was a great learning experience. It was my privilege to see him save a life. Following a long morning in the operating room, my father and I were putting on our coats to leave when a woman struggled through the outside door and collapsed on the floor in front of us. With the supervisor's help, we lifted her onto a stretcher. She told us there had been no foetal movement for a couple weeks. She had just passed some clots, tissue, and was bleeding heavily. Obviously, she was spontaneously aborting a four- to five-month foetus. We raced her to the operating room where the nursing staff were already scrubbing and opening packs. Intravenous lines were inserted, and plasma and other volume expanders started, in an effort to replace her rapid loss of blood. Unfortunately, our small hospital had not been granted the privilege of stocking blood so we would have to wait for it to arrive from the outside depot. We knew removal of the remaining tissue, which was preventing the uterus from contracting, should control the bleeding. This could not wait. Dad quickly had the patient asleep, and I carefully emptied the uterus, grateful for my postgraduate surgical training. Even when empty, the uterus remained flaccid, and the bleeding continued. Near toxic doses of medications were administered and the volume expanders continued. I re-examined the uterine cavity and found it clean with no damage to the muscle. The uterus stubbornly refused to contract despite manual stimulation and pressure.

I told my father, "I'm afraid of losing her . . . I don't know what more I can do . . . I can't control the bleeding."

He told me to continue, got up, passed the maintenance of the anaesthetic to the nurse, and, cupping one fist over the other, leaned over the patient's abdomen, pressing hard enough to occlude the aorta. The bleeding stopped immediately. After a short period of time the uterus responded to the medications and began to contract, allowing dad to relax his pressure. There was no further bleeding and he returned to the anaesthetic. Without question he saved the woman's life.

During my first years in practice, I gained obstetrical experience doing deliveries for patients whose doctors were unavailable. On one such occasion, I received a call from the hospital asking me to come immediately for a delivery. The supervisor admitted she knew the attending physician was home because he had answered the phone, but his only response was snoring. His phone was now off the hook, she could not call him back, and the labour was progressing rapidly. I was needed immediately, and I went. The next morning, I reviewed the delivery with the physician in question, who sheepishly apologized and confessed he had woken that morning with the phone still buzzing next to his ear. His only memory of the night was the supervisor's voice saying, "Oh, shit." He was still wondering what he had missed.

I was sympathetic, as I remembered waking one night standing in my driveway, my back turned toward the biting night wind, fully dressed in my winter coat and boots. Why was I there? Was I dreaming? I was fully dressed, medical bag in one gloved hand, car keys in the other. Was there an urgent house call; if so, where? Possibly I was needed at a hospital, but which one? Or had I already made the visit? Was I on my way home to bed? Puzzled, I went back into the house and called WKMH. They had not called; I was not needed there. I noticed concern for my wellbeing in their comments: Was I okay? Did I need help? Hesitantly, I called Soldiers Memorial Hospital and was told the obstetric team was anxiously awaiting my arrival. The labour was progressing more rapidly than usual. As I had not yet left, they would ask Dr. Kelley to stand by until I arrived.

As I entered Kingston village, any lingering drowsiness disappeared when a deer jumped over the hood of the car. Neither the car, the deer, nor I was injured. Upon my arrival at the hospital, Dr. Kelly went home with the patient's and my thanks. I had the pleasure of delivering a healthy infant.

As the practice grew, it impinged on family time, and even on my mealtimes, especially lunch. My routine workday became giving anaesthetics in the morning; racing home for a quick noon meal; afternoon office appointments which often went late; and after the evening meal, a return to the hospital for pre-op assessments. Lunch I made a priority, even if patients early for their appointments were waiting in my home office. One noontime, my wife told me there was a woman waiting who should be seen immediately, even before I had lunch. Entering the office, I was met by a plump, middle-aged-appearing patient pacing up and down and complaining of constipation. Surely this could have waited until after my lunch, I thought, but it was unusual to see this woman unaccompanied by both her father and mother, with whom she resided and who usually spoke for her. Making an exception from my usual policy of not examining a patient without a third person present, I asked her to lie down on the examining table. She refused, saying she was in too much pain. I countered with, "How can I tell what is causing the pain if you won't let me examine you?" Finally, after much back-and-forth of "I need to examine you," and her reply, "It hurts too much to lie down," and with my stomach rumbling, I gave in and sent her to the hospital outpatient department for the requested enema. I began my lunch only to have another interruption. This time it was the hospital supervisor informing me with a snicker, "Doctor, your patient is ready to deliver."

I never lived down that particular diagnosis; and never did get my lunch.

Nighttime

One evening in the fall of 1963, I counted a hundred bats in just a few short minutes, emerging from under the shingles of the home I had just acquired. As we went to bed a few evenings later, we were greeted by a bat flying wildly around the bedroom. My frantic efforts to capture it and put it outside were unsuccessful. We were so tired we crawled into bed, ignoring our visitor. It was still there the next day, resting in an inaccessible location. With no easy way to catch the bat, I searched an encyclopedia, hoping to find a safe removal method and found this suggestion: *Wait for night, put on lights in the adjacent room, but leave the room containing the bat in darkness. Then open the window. The bat, with its fear of light, would use its radar to find a way outside, through the open window to freedom.* Revelling in my newfound knowledge, I did just that. To my disappointment and surprise, another bat had joined the first and the two kept flying into each other. So much for bat radar. With the return of daylight, I was able to locate both and put them outside, to the relief of all concerned.

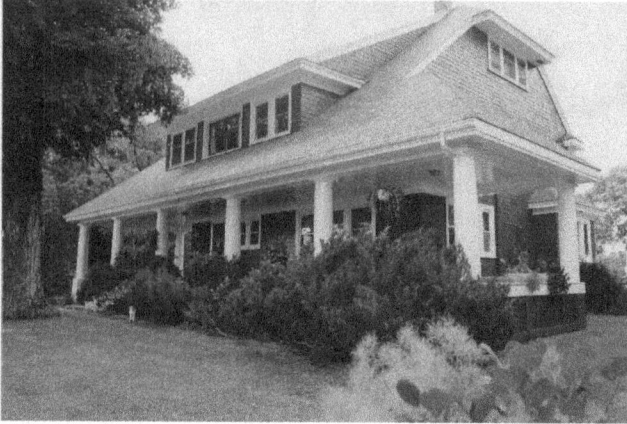

My house in Aylesford where I had the basement renovated for my Practice.

I recounted my story in the doctors' change room, and that prompted Dr. Paul Kinsman to tell us of his bat adventure. The previous night his mother had woken him, screaming that there was a bat in her bedroom. Going to her rescue, he trapped the creature on the window screen and drugged it using chloroform from his obstetrical bag. Paul, like most other doctors at that time, had a special kit ready for home deliveries and other emergencies. It was public knowledge that our medical bags contained chloroform, ether, narcotics and other drugs, but I never heard of a theft. My father knew our community was so secure and honest that car keys were always in the ignition of his unattended cars, his medical bag on the back seat. Day or night, he was ready for any emergency. His only loss to theft in all his years in practice was a blanket one cold winter night.

Somewhat later in my medical practice, I received a telephone request from a caller asking to buy ether. I explained I no longer had any, as newer and better agents had replaced its use. Curious, I asked why he needed the ether. Apparently, his dog had caught a porcupine and its mouth and face were now full of quills. The dog would have to be put asleep if the quills were to be removed. I suggested he call the hospital, explain his plight, and if they had any left in stock they might, possibly, sell him a small amount. Then he asked me how to use it. I explained he could take a preserving ring, cover it with several layers of gauze, and place this over the dog's nose. Next, he should cautiously put a few drops of ether in a pattern on the gauze, continuing to add more until the dog was asleep. He should be extremely careful not to get any of the irritating ether in the dog's eyes. Having thought this over, the caller confessed he had been using pliers to remove the quills and the dog would no longer let him near him. My next suggestion was one I had witnessed my father using: confine the dog with a sponge soaked in ether, under an inverted wooden box. When the dog ceased struggling, he most likely would be asleep. Another thoughtful pause, then: "Would you do it? I am afraid he will bite." I refused, but suggested he go to a veterinary doctor. The answer was: "Oh the dog is not worth a vet . . . they are too expensive . . . you are cheaper." I hung up the phone, not asking or even wanting to know what finally happened to the unfortunate dog.

We all had unexpected night visits. Everyone in the community knew where the doctors and the nurses lived, and when they were worried, we were easily found.

One night, insistent ringing of my doorbell accompanied by heavy pounding and shaking of the front door, awakened the whole household, including me. Somehow the door lock was rattled loose. Still getting out of bed, I now heard the intruder coming up the stairs yelling "Doctor . . . Doctor . . . Doctor . . ."

I barely managed to contain him at my bedroom door as he approached, yelling, "I just saw an unconscious man on the street. This is an emergency! He's probably dead! You must go at once!"

"Where?" I asked.

"That way!" he said, pointing to the west.

I asked him to guide me to the injured man because I might require his help.

He refused, saying he was "too scared." This was "the first dead man he had ever seen." It would be impossible for me to miss the man, as he was lying on the road. Refusing to leave until he saw me in my car, he then went home to bed. I was left to drive in the direction of what I guessed was the area indicated. Arriving at what I presumed to be the disaster location, a thorough search did not reveal anything unusual. Even the surrounding landscape appeared undisturbed. Apparently the "Good Samaritan" had not seen his first fatality. The dead man had either revived or had been resuscitated. I was no longer needed, and I, too, went home to bed.

The following morning, I discussed my adventure in the doctor's room, as I was wondering if one of the other doctors had dealt with the casualty. None had, and all of the physicians except me had slept peacefully that night. We surmised there was someone else who, like me, had not slept well, but unlike me, was nursing a severe hangover.

My story prompted Dr. MacArthur to share one of his nighttime episodes. He began by saying he wished the location of his sleeping area was like mine, on the second floor of the house. My staircase and its distance from the entrance door had delayed the intruder in my home, allowing me to confront him and prevent him from entering my bedroom. Mac's intruder had no such delay, as there was easy access to his ground floor bedroom from his outside entrance. His first realization of a third party in his bedroom was being shaken by someone yelling, "Wake up! Wake up!" Soon he realized the bedclothes were being yanked off his and his wife's scantily-clad bodies, and there then began a tug of war—the panicked man trying to pull the sheets off the couple, yelling, "Get up, get up," the nearly naked couple pulling back on the bedclothes, yelling, "Get out, get out."

The invader turned out to be a first-time father who had raced his wife to the hospital the instant her labour began. Once she had been admitted, he was told the doctor would be informed and called when needed. The panicked man wanted the doctor there right away and had rushed to his house to rouse him.

My grandfather, like all country doctors, had his full share of emergency night calls. Prominent in his memory was a trip that took him into a fierce winter storm one night in 1906, his first year in practice. Dr. Covert, an older physician living in Canning who was employed by the Federal Government as the local First Nation's doctor, had requested grandfather make the call. In better weather Dr. Covert would have made the visit himself, but he did not feel able to face the raging storm and had called Grandfather, a younger doctor living closer to the Mi'kmaq, to go to the reservation in his stead. Grandfather immediately readied his horse and sleigh and went out into the storm, knowing only that "they were all upset and worried about something." The dim golden glow of oil-lamp-lit windows announced his arrival at the village. The light reflecting off the snow revealed a group of men waiting for him. The welcoming committee were all snugly wrapped in warm clothing against the cold and blowing snow. They took his horse and sleigh to a shelter, and him to the door of one of the small homes, where he was abandoned. No one would accompany him inside.

Alone, he opened the door to find a small room with beds crowded together, containing people heavily wrapped in blankets. To keep them warm, their beds were closely arranged around a red-hot, pot-bellied stove. All appeared to be very sick and to have high fevers. The single oil lamp was thick with soot and provided very little light. Removing his gloves, Grandfather pulled back the blankets of the nearest patient, leaned in close with the lamp in his hands, trying to see enough to make a diagnosis in the almost-dark room. There was a rash. He bent closer, his face almost touching the rash, to do his examination. Suddenly he realized it was smallpox, to which he was now exposed.

Grandfather had always tried to avoid exposure to smallpox knowing he had no immunity to the disease. His vaccinations in childhood had not taken, neither had the two subsequent vaccinations he had received during his medical school days. In 1796 Dr.

Edward Jenner observed that milkmaids often had cowpox but rarely had smallpox. He surmised that infection with cowpox gave protection to smallpox as well. He tested his assertion by infecting an 8-year-old boy with cowpox and found the child developed immunity to both cowpox and smallpox. The procedure for smallpox vaccination was to use a needle to break the skin only in one spot through which the virus was introduced. If a pustule appeared in 3 to 4 days the vaccination took, and there was immunity. If nothing developed, then it had not taken and there was no immunity. Grandfather had now been intimately exposed and was not protected from the frequently fatal disease. If he became infected there was a high risk some of his family members would also develop the illness. Still, since his exposure had already occurred, he decided he had nothing more to lose. Driven by curiosity, he proceeded to carefully examine the patient and the rash. After doing what little he could for the sick, he returned home.

Upon his arrival home, standing on the open veranda in the blowing snow, he removed all his clothes. Leaving them outside, he proceeded naked to his home office where he very carefully vaccinated himself. He knew the incubation period for smallpox was seven to seventeen days; the incubation period needed for his vaccination to prevent smallpox to "take," would be four to seven days. If he was fortunate and his self-vaccination took, he might possibly avoid the illness. Mercifully, it took, and both he and his family were spared. He burned his clothes to be certain they would not contaminate anyone. There had been no smallpox in Nova Scotia for several years prior to this 1906 smallpox epidemic, which eventually involved some 1,860 cases. In subsequent years, sporadic cases from outside the province were quarantined in seaports. He had been asked to diagnose some of these because of his knowledge of the disease.

My father also had many night calls. We children only vaguely realized how tired he was after being up all night. We played noisily in the living room while he slept in his leather chair. He wanted to be there, with us, and so he was not disturbed by our activities. Mother was protective and tried to keep our din under control to allow him to sleep. She, however, said she always resented one of the night calls he had received during a severe snowstorm. He was requested to go to the home of a new patient to conduct her first delivery. He got up, shovelled out his car, and with quite an effort managed to get to the home in question. Arriving at the door, he was greeted by the husband in his nightclothes with, "Don't bother coming in, she is not in labour. We just wanted to see if you would come during weather like this when she actually does go into labour."

My mother was angry with the patient, but she was just as annoyed at our father because he returned to conduct the actual delivery when the patient's true labour began.

During a coffee break from a long meeting, I was speaking with a Department of Health official. He indicated the department was considering paying only for "medically necessary home visits." In an effort to illustrate the difficulty of determining the medical necessity of a visit prior to preforming an actual examination, I told him about a recent call I had received.

Near midnight one evening, I stopped for gas at a twenty-four-hour service station on my way home to bed. A grandfather, also there for fuel, approached me with his grandson on his arm. The son and grandson were my patients, but not the grandparents themselves. I had just discharged the convalescing child from hospital and was tempted to chastise the senior for keeping him out so late, but I bit my tongue and went home to bed. I had been asleep about thirty minutes when the phone rang. It was the child's grandmother who said her husband asked her to call me to come, for he had a cold. I could have suggested they call their own doctor; I could have told her he had no complaints when we had been speaking a few minutes before, or I could have sent them to the hospital outpatient department for treatment. I am grateful that despite my semi-awake state I said I would come immediately. He was dead when I arrived and could not be resuscitated.

How can anyone accurately and safely always predict which night calls, or even which house calls were medically necessary, prior to examining the patient? I confess I cannot, and I doubt if others are more clairvoyant than I.

Carriage Rug

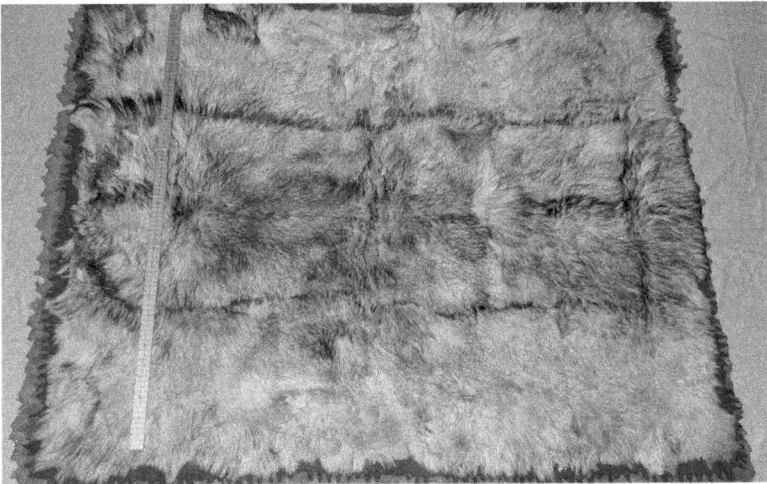

A wolf fur rug was gifted by the local Mi'kmaq community to my grandfather Harold, after he broke his hip in a carriage accident. A staff member at the Hudson's Bay Archives in Winnipeg told us that their collection of over 150,000 items did not include anything similar. (Note the Meter stick for size)
Cogswell Photo

As children, we knew the Mi'kmaq had given a "Bear Rug" to Grandfather Killam. We rarely saw it, as it smelled too much like the barn for the living room, having been used outdoors in the wagon and sleigh. The rug was stored with the winter clothing in the unheated entrance foyer of the house. Occasionally, if we arrived unexpectedly, we found Grandfather warmly snuggled under it in his chair. Grandma would quickly return it to the storage area, apologizing that the blanket must smell of horse and barn. After my mother inherited the rug, she continued the tradition of keeping the "dirty" blanket stored away from the living area. The carriage rug had been presented to Grandfather by the First Nations people following an accident in 1931 when he was fifty-three years old. His skittish horse had spooked, bolted, and overturned the wagon leaving him on the ground with a fractured hip.

Carriage rugs were used to augment buffalo rugs during cold winter sleigh rides, as clearly shown in Krieghoff paintings[9], and only the best furs were utilized. This rug is so beautiful and unusual that I showed it to Carol Harris[10], academic and dog lover. She noticed it smelled like dog, and believed it was most likely was wolf, as others had suggested. Karen Diadick Casselman, PhD.[11], an authority on weaving and dyes, identified the fabric backing as handspun and handwoven wool, dyed with natural dyes of a type in use circa 1880. She noted the edging was similarly composed of handwoven, felted wool, also coloured with natural dyes.

Intrigued, she and I sought another opinion from Sharon MacDonald[12], who is the author of books and papers on quilts and hooked mats. Sharon considered it outside her area of expertise but during her years doing museum research had never seen this style of rug.

Next, we consulted Ruth Holmes[13] Whitehead, a leading expert on Mi'kmaq material culture. She, too, had never seen such a rug. As there were no wolves in Nova Scotia, she felt it was likely to have been brought here as a trade item. Ruth noted that the fringed edging on the rug was like the edging commonly used to decorate the sleeves, leggings and other areas of Mi'kmaq and Métis clothing. This feature can also be seen in Krieghoff paintings[14]. She cautioned us that identifying the age of the rug might be difficult, as First Nations peoples had few processions and carefully reused and recycled materials, making it possible that each component of our rug, the fabric backing, the fringes, and even the fur, could have a different date of origin.

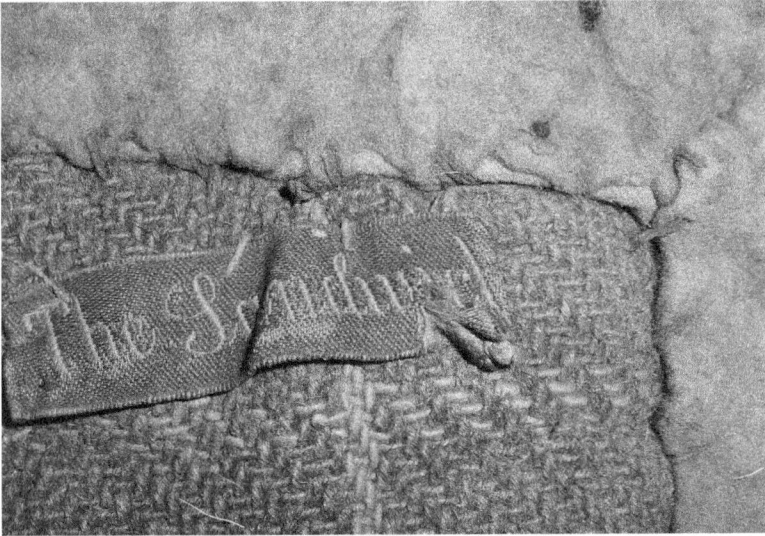

Label, "The Sandwich" on the rug.
Photo: David Cogswell

With the passage of time, the rug has become more mysterious. Despite the consultations, everyone missed a crucial detail: there is a label on the rug. It says simply "The Sandwich," its origin or meaning one that no one, as yet, can explain.

Grandfather especially prized two gifts he had received following his accident: the rug from the Mi'kmaq and a lazy-boy chair given to him by the community as a sign of their respect and sympathy. The chair, "Grandfather's chair," is long gone. The sleigh rug remains in good condition, its origin, its history, even the label "The Sandwich," still an incomprehensible mystery.

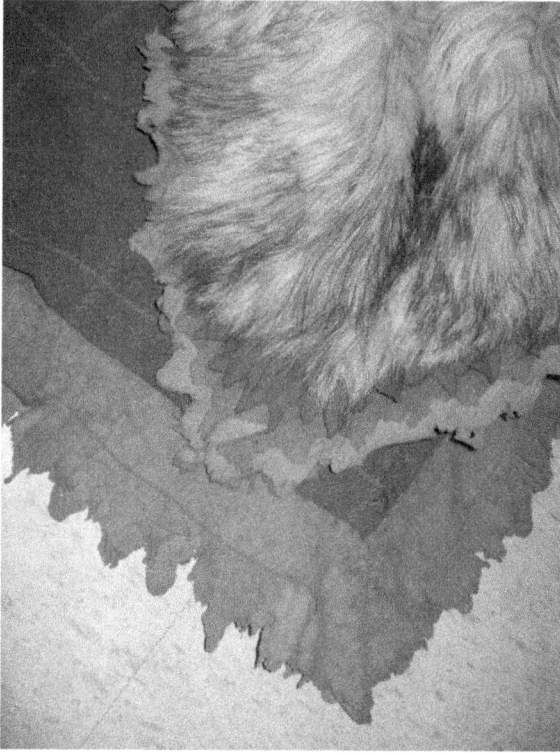

Carriage Rug of Wolf Fur, from First Nation
Cogswell Photo

Morden

During the early years of my practice, communities were frequently isolated by snowstorms, and 1965 was one of those years. The snowfalls had been frequent and heavy, and drifting snow blocked roads opened only hours earlier by the Department of Highways plows. They had difficulty keeping the main road in front of my house open. The private company clearing my yard returned frequently to allow me to reach the hospital and deal with emergencies. Now a lull between storms permitted snowplows to open secondary roads to communities that had been isolated for days, The banks of snow in places were so high parents were afraid their children, while climbing on top of them, might touch the power lines carrying high-voltage electricity. We all worried that children who were making tunnels in drifts on the side of the road might be struck by subsequent snowplows when they returned to widen the roads. These drifts were deeper on the mountain roads where the snowfall was greater.

I received a call that someone in Morden, on the Bay of Fundy, was very sick and had been getting worse daily. The road to the community had been impassable for over a week, isolating the community. Plows had just opened a one-lane track from the valley over the mountain and into the village, but the storm was filling it in rapidly. Would I come at once and see the sick, while the road was still passable? I should take Long Point, the only mountain road open. The Harbourville, Aylesford, Morden, and Kingston mountain roads had not been plowed and were not passable. Dressing warmly, taking all drug samples and other things I might need, off I went. I got up Long Point without difficulty, but when I reached the top and turned west, there were whiteouts and drifts forming in the road, with high banks of snow on either side.

When I arrived at the village, warmly dressed residents were waiting to take me to the patient, whom I examined and gave sample meds. I was prepared to leave for home before the falling snow again blocked the road when a number of other sick people appeared anxious to be seen as well. As soon as they were seen, others took their place. I suddenly realized I was now seeing people the weather had prevented from attending their usual routine doctor appointments.

As quickly as possible I completed my impromptu clinic, rushed to my car and started it, but before I could leave, the back door was pulled open. "I'm going with you," I'm too scared to stay here", a woman said as she jumped into the back seat. I asked where in the valley would she stay, and she said she didn't care, she wasn't staying in Morden. Her family tried to calm her panic and gradually they were able to reassure her that the road would remain open even though it continued to snow. She lost her look of anxiety, got out of my car, and I was off home alone, probably more anxious than she. The snowdrifts across the one-lane plowed mountain road had become more pronounced. To break through these barriers, I accelerated when the road was relatively clear, then hit each drift, which sent snow up over the hood and windshield. The momentum carried the car through. I trusted the banks of snow on either side to keep me on the road. The trip down the mountain was uneventful, and soon I was safely back in the valley and headed west towards home.

Following paths made by previous vehicles through the snowdrifts, I came to a stretch of highway blown free of snow beyond which was a large drift blocking the road, with an abandoned car stuck in the middle, completely blocking the road. I could go no further. I moved my car to the side of the open area, leaving enough space for a snowplow to go around it, put the key in the ignition, and walked the distance to my friend Allen's house. Allen drove me home, and later, after the plow had cleared the road, he walked to my car and brought it to me.

My sleep was broken later that night when I was called to the hospital to see a snowplow operator, by coincidence the one who had plowed out my car earlier that evening. He had left the security of the interior of the plow to make some adjustments when a fierce gust of wind had driven the door against his head causing a lot of damage to his ear. I kept him in hospital for observation overnight and repaired it the next day under general anaesthesia; my father gave the anaesthetic. He made a good recovery.

Office Interruptions

The most frequent interruptions to my office appointments were from the hospital, but local events intervened as well; some were medical and some not.

Intersection Collision

One afternoon a man rushed into my consultation room announcing I was urgently needed outside. I grabbed my medical bag. As we ran, we heard the blare of the village fire alarm calling its volunteer members, which signaled that this was a serious accident. A truck and van had collided in the intersection near my home office. The driver's side of the van had sustained the most damage. I entered the vehicle through the rear door to find the driver pinned to his seat by the doorpost, dash, and steering wheel. Making a careful assessment of his injuries and examining the manner in which he was trapped by the debris, I decided how to protect him during his rescue. Only then did I begin to look for the cause of the hissing sound I had previously ignored, assuming it was air escaping from a tire. But now I realized this was a delivery truck full of oxygen and acetylene tanks on route to various welding shops. Damaged by the impact of the accident, gas was escaping from one or more of these tanks. One spark and the whole lot would explode, destroying the truck, the driver, and myself as well as the centre of the village. It was urgent to get the driver outside as quickly as possible.

A tap on my shoulder and a "Doc, can I help you?" caught me by surprise. I had not heard anyone enter the vehicle. I turned around, expecting to see a fireman. Instead, I saw a man in a cloud of smoke, puffing on a cigarette. In fear and horror, I yelled, "YES, TAKE THAT CIGARETTE AND GET THE HELL OUT OF HERE!"

He left, to be replaced by a volunteer fireman—a welder by profession—who efficiently stopped the gas leak and made it safe to release the driver from his imprisonment. The injured driver was taken to hospital for treatment. We all survived.

KLM Flight

During a flight from Halifax to Germany to visit Heide's family, my reverie was broken when "Is there a doctor on board?" came over the speakers. I hesitated to answer, hoping another physician more familiar with the international names of drugs, and the management of airline emergences, would appear. After the third request, I identified myself. As the stewardess escorted me to the first-class section, we passed a man who looked both worried and relieved; was he a specialist physician uncomfortable with acute emergencies, or just a relieved passenger, I wondered? The patient, an older woman dressed in black, was pressing both hands to her chest. There was fear in her eyes. Was she was having a heart attack, or unstable angina, or a hiatus hernia, or was this a panic attack? I began asking her medical history, as the stewardess handed me a stethoscope. The patient rebuffed my attempt to do an examination and made no effort to respond to my questioning, even though she seemed to know I was speaking to her. I asked if she was deaf and was told she only understood Greek. Hoping for a translator, I asked the stewardess to find out if someone on board spoke Greek. I did not hear the broadcast, but when I returned to my seat, Heide and the other passengers heard her request, "Is there a doctor on board who speaks Greek?" No wonder there was no response.

Without any history and without any real examination, I needed to make an accurate diagnosis and then decide where she would receive the best care. The plane was halfway across the ocean, and I asked myself if it was more reasonable for the flight to continue to Europe, or was the woman sufficiently at risk for me to recommend we return to Halifax? I asked to see the airline's medical kit so I would know what emergency equipment and medications were available. This was grudgingly produced by the stewardess, who complained that this would cause her more paperwork.

I spent the remainder of the flight going back and forth monitoring the patient. After we landed, she was taken off the plane by stretcher. I was no longer needed and was ignored. We were the last off the flight. This had not been the relaxed journey I had envisaged.

RCMP Parking

Parking is a problem everywhere. My office provided more than enough space for patients coming to their appointments. If I was delayed by an emergency and those six spaces were occupied, overflow parking was available in front of my house or across the road. My personal parking spot was obvious: the carport attached to the house. This was clearly mine and freed me to come and go as necessary.

Returning late one day, I found the yard full, and in addition, an RCMP squad car had squeezed into the carport. I parked in one of the free spaces on the street and entered the office. Before I could speak with my receptionist, two RCMP officers presented me with a summons to be an expert witness. I had been required to do this previously, and it was a task I did not enjoy. I was surprised that the police had commandeered my dedicated parking space and then had appeared unannounced in my office. I also found it unsettling to be presented with a summons in front of a waiting room full of murmuring patients.

The police left, their task completed, only to abruptly return. This time they asked to speak to me in private. Once in the quiet of the consulting room, they admitted that in their rush to leave, the side of the patrol car had come up against one of the carport pillars, damaging both the car and pillar. The visit and the damage were annoying, but I had difficulty not looking smug.

Patient Parking

On another occasion my office was interrupted by a pedestrian looking for the owner of a car that was obstructing the sidewalk in front of my house. We found the owner, and I accompanied her outside. Her vehicle was across the sidewalk, the back wheels high up on the lawn embankment in front of my house, the grill and bumper jammed against a power pole. We were astounded. The driverless car had coasted from where she had originally parked, in my busy office parking-lot, down through the empty carport, and landed where it now was, completely unscathed. In this journey down my lawn, the car had somehow missed my ornamental light-post. How fortunate the power pole had stopped the car. Otherwise, the vehicle would have continued moving, driverless, across the busy highway and into the restaurant parking lot on the other side of the road, hitting anything or anybody in its path.

The owner of the vehicle was incredulous. She insisted my office parking area was defective. She assured me her car (the first she had owned with an automatic transmission), had been parked in gear and could not therefore, be at fault. She always left her cars parked in gear and had never engaged or needed to engage the emergency brake. She continued this habit with the new car, always leaving it parked in "D," in "Drive," in gear. The group of onlookers gradually convinced her that leaving an automatic transmission in "D" was the same as leaving her previous cars in neutral. She learned that an automatic transmission should be left in "P" when parked, "Park" and the parking brake both should always be used. It seemed to me a miracle that this vehicle, regularly parked in "Drive," had not coasted away before this and had not injured or killed anyone, and how little damage had resulted from its present adventure.

Car Wreck Blocking Driveway

I returned home from the hospital one evening to find my driveway and the surrounding highway full of police cars, ambulances, fire trucks, and people. There were flashing lights everywhere. Medical bag in hand, fearing the worst, I dashed toward the center of attention, which was an overturned car in the entrance to my driveway. Thankfully my family was safe watching the spectacle on the lawn, not injured in the accident. Fire trucks were spreading foam to prevent the whole scene from exploding into flames. The smell of gasoline overpowered everything. Teams of people were struggling to gain entrance to the wreck, the wheels in the air, still spinning. The roof and the windows of the vehicle had been driven completely into the body of the car.

The massive destruction of the vehicle elicited from me, "I guess I'm not needed here. I can't see how anyone could still be alive in this mess."

From inside the wreck came a voice, "I'm still alive! Help! Get me out of here!"

Later, we learned the driver had been upset, was speeding, lost control of his vehicle and left the road to careen along the embankment at the foot of my lawn. Despite being slowed by hitting and destroying shrubs, the car, on reaching my driveway, had somersaulted and ended up on its roof. The lucky driver had been thrown to the safety of the car's floor by the rotation; the roof had become his floor. It took some time to extricate him from the wreckage. Amazingly, he sustained only moderate injuries.

Tree Blocking Driveway

I enjoyed stormy days. My office was in the house so when appointments were missed, I was home and could catch up on paperwork, or if school was cancelled, I had time with my family.

This present storm seemed different. Despite the high winds and steady rain, there were no cancellations. I asked one elderly patient how she'd managed to arrive for her appointment in such bad weather. Did a neighbour bring her?

"I wanted to try out my new four-wheel-drive truck," was her response. Times were changing.

The wind and rain still raging outside, I finished with my last patient and entered the waiting room. To my surprise, everyone I had seen that afternoon was still there, sitting politely and visiting with each other. They had been unable to leave. A large maple tree had been uprooted and was now blocking my driveway, trapping their vehicles in my yard. My day was not over. With my chainsaw, I removed enough branches to fashion a tunnel under the tree, through which they all left. We had a late supper, and office was cancelled until professionals cleaned up the mess.

Vignettes

As interns, we were required to give injections of any medications known to be painful or have possible unpleasant local side effects. With our lack of experience in giving injections, we relied on senior nursing staff for guidance. I considered my technique polished, having been taught under supervision during my summer "Junior Internship" at the Sanatorium, only to have classmate Otto teach me there is a psychological component to any procedure.

Otto was given a tray by the medication nurse and sent to give Mrs. XYZ her intramuscular injection. When she saw him go in the wrong direction, the nurse realized there were two patients with the same surname, and he was headed towards the wrong one. She raced after him. But by the time she had caught up, the patient was on her side, back to the door, hip exposed, ready for the injection. Otto, syringe in hand, was ready to proceed. The nurse jumped up and down vigorously and shook her head to get his attention. Seeing her antics, Otto calmly placed the unused syringe back on the tray, wiped her bottom with another alcohol swab, and announced, "There! I told you wouldn't feel a thing."

Accent

To appear professional, I tried not to use local colloquialisms such as "out-n-about" or "some-good" when away from home but did not realize I had an accent until I was in a campground in Germany.

Exiting our tent I was admiring the Porsche sportscar parked opposite us. I noted its oval number plate indicating it was for export and greeted the owner with "hi" instead of "Guten Tag" as he approached me.

"Did you say hi?" he exclaimed.

His wife, hearing us, came out of their elaborate tent, introduced herself and joined the English conversation. Abruptly she looked at me and said, "You are from Nova Scotia!" Then added, "With that accent you must live somewhere within thirty miles of Port Williams."

Her home had been in Port Williams until her marriage, and she recognized an accent I always denied having.

When I was home, during a weekend break from my resident training, I stopped for a drink of water from a mountain spring near the town of Berwick. Locals often came here to collect their drinking water to take home. A stranger struck up a conversation with me and asked where I was from.

"Berwick," I answered.

"Not with that accent," was his retort. "But I just can't quite place it. Where are you from?" My accent was recognized in Germany, but not in my home town.

German English Class

On one of my visits to Germany I was invited to the local school to participate in their English class. Afterwards, the teacher thanked me as he escorted me politely out of the school. At the door he said, authoritatively, "Of course we know your English is not correct English."

I replied that I considered my English excellent. I had my Medical Degree, as did my father, and my mother, with her master's degree, taught English. What mistakes had he found?

He replied, "The only correct pronunciation of English is that spoken by the Queen—the 'Queen's English.' You do not sound like her."

I am afraid he returned to the class and told them my English was incorrect; could it have been my accent.

Canadian Council
on Health Services
Accreditation (CCHSA)

Sitting in my office one afternoon in 1993, I realized that my solo country practice caused me to miss out on the daily informal contacts my colleagues—who worked in larger community group practices—had with each other. Practicing alone did not provide the opportunity for casual discussions about how new therapies or even social events were changing our medical lives, nor did I have anyone to whom I could compare myself. Our hospital had just been visited by the Canadian Council on Health Services Accreditation (CCHSA) surveyors, and I had observed how well their team functioned. I spoke to the doctor on the team, who encouraged me to join. I realized it would be an interesting and useful organization to join; it would keep me up to date about health care, I would see how medicine was practiced in other areas of Canada, and might even be sent to Bermuda, which was part of the Canadian Service.

I knew that CCHSA was independent of both the medical society and the government. This "arm's length" structure was so effective that each thought it was a branch of the other. CCHSA had its origins in the USA, when a surgeon determined that his profession could access his degree of competency, but there was no organization that reviewed hospitals. How could he know what was excellent or what was problematic in the hospitals where he worked? An educational organization free of outside pressures was needed, and the American Hospital Accreditation was established. Standards of excellence applicable to any hospital were developed, with peer surveyors trained to review hospitals. Those meeting the standard received Accreditation. A hospital in Yarmouth, Nova Scotia was the first in Canada to be reviewed by the American Accreditation program. This American venture became so successful that a Canadian version evolved. The American system had, and has, full time surveyors. In Canada, surveyors are required to be in full-time practice.

I applied to be a medical surveyor, was accepted, and went for my training at head office in Ottawa. Arriving there, I was first introduced to the staff, two of whom enthusiastically said, "We told them to accept you." They were previous patients of mine, and now we were working as colleagues. Following the basic office training, I was sent on a survey with an experienced medical surveyor to gain some practical experience. We discussed our findings and how we should deal with them each evening. He did the official report; mine was critiqued by head office. I learned a great deal during that first survey. Coincidentally, this same hospital was also the last one I surveyed prior to my retirement in 2003.

Smaller hospitals, similar to those I had worked in all my professional life, were my survey expertise. They usually required one medical and one nurse surveyor, although some slightly larger hospitals required a third surveyor, an administrator. I was very fortunate to be paired with excellent nurses who taught me a great deal. The small hospitals I surveyed tended to be in remote areas, and I was never sure of what I would find. On one occasion I knew we would be travelling on a water taxi and decided to take casual clothes as well as my suit, boots instead of office footwear, and fly repellent. The nurse arrived wearing a skirt and dress shoes with spike heels. In the time we were waiting for the water taxi, she became covered in blackflies. We had also arrived in pouring rain. The path to the two buildings that constituted the "hospital complex" was muddy, and she sank in up to her ankles. By the time we reached the residence my boots were covered, as were her ankles and feet. Her dress shoes were ruined. Inside the door were rubber boots the doctors and nurses used for their walks to the hospital. They carried their shoes. We both borrowed rubber boots and were given slippers, which enabled us to do the survey. A proper walkway was one of our recommendations.

On another survey, a six-passenger plane landed us in a remote community where the only connection to the outside during the summer was by air, and these flights only occurred three days a week. I had been told a previous surveyor team had been late for their flight home, missed it, and had to remain in the community a couple of days longer for the next flight out, so I knew how important timing was going to be over the next couple of days. The hospital was well organized and made full use of our time during the survey. Following our final sum-up meeting, the questions continued, and time was passing. I voiced my concerns and was reassured the plane would wait for us, as we were the only passengers. With no apparent end to the questioning, I abruptly ended the session, and we left in a rush. We watched our incoming plane land from our taxi. Upon reaching the airport, we were rushed onboard the plane which immediately took off; we had nearly missed our flight.

Surveyors came from all across the country, so team members usually did not know one another unless they had met during a previous survey. This anonymity protected us as surveyors, and also the hospitals. Not knowing each other's strengths and weaknesses, and with so little time to form a team, we tried to find each other in the airport and get to know each other on the flight to the hospital. We wore our name tags and scanned the departure lounge for someone wearing the same identification. At that time, the majority of doctors were male, and most nurses were female. A survey team was generally comprised of one of each so I would look around for women who appeared to be on their own, then go closer to check for a name tag. Sometimes I met my team partner, while at other times all I got was an indignant stare.

Accreditation reviews occurred in five-year intervals and were designed to help all hospital staff members upgrade and improve. The hospitals were provided with extensive documentation against which they could measure their own performance. There were specific recommendations for each department—from janitorial to surgical—which were constantly being upgraded. We, as surveyors, reviewed the hospitals, their procedures, medical records, and facilities. We found and gave suggestions to help deal with problem areas. We inspected the hospitals from the emergency generator, kitchen, and patient rooms to the operating theatres. Having prepared for the survey team's visit during the five-year interval between surveys, staff could be quite anxious when interviewed, whether one-on-one or as part of a group, as all wanted their hospital to be Accredited. At times their efforts surprised us. We began the survey by reviewing and following the signage to the hospitals. Arriving at a hospital on one occasion, we saw beds and other equipment being loaded on trucks. We asked why they were doing this and were told there were important people coming; the truckers had been hired to remove excess beds and other clutter from the halls and return them in four days, after the inspectors were gone.

On another occasion, in a picturesque village in Newfoundland, we three surveyors drove in circles following the signage trying to find the hospital, which, to our chagrin, when found, was the only multi-storey building in the community.

There often was a sense of relief mixed with excitement when the surveys were completed; it would be five years before their next review. One nurse/administrator I worked with, told of opening a large refrigerator during one of her kitchen reviews. Due to her height, she saw a cake hidden on the top shelf in a corner. She asked why the cake was there and was told they did not know there was a cake. Awkwardly reaching in, she pulled out the cake with "Thank God They Are Gone" written in the frosting.

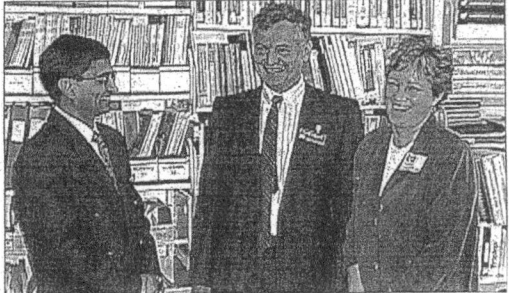

FCHS opens its doors for voluntary evaluation

Paul Mayne
The Chronicle

Four Counties Health Services have once again opened its doors to accreditation inspectors to ensure the community that all services and program at the hospital are functioning at a acceptable levels.

The last survey conducted by the Canadian Council on Health Services Accreditation (CCHSA) at FCHS in 1995, resulted in a three-year accreditation for the hospital.

The voluntary accreditation survey provides the hospital an opportunity to be evaluated by an independent, non-governmental agency. The major focus is on how care is provided and communicated to the patient from a team perspective during the patient's episode of care within the hospital.

Surveyors Dr. David Cogswell, a family practitioner in the village of Aylesford, Nova Scotia (pop. 1,000) and Heather Klein-Swormink, vice-president of FCHS with staff members that were organized into five teams including:

✔ Leadership and Partnership
✔ Human Resources and Information Management
✔ Environmental Management
✔ Inpatient Care Team
✔ Outpatient Care Team

The teams were made up of members of the community, volunteers and front-line staff from all departments, department managers, physicians and board members. Team members spent the past two years working together to identify and determine ways to meet the needs of the community.

During difficult economic times, hospital administrator Janak Jass realizes this is a vital process to assess performance against a set of nationally applied standards, to assure that services provided by the hospital meet acceptable standards and to focus on ways to continuously improve service.

"With all the restructuring and funding restrictions this is a good test for us to make sure we are still meeting, or exceeding, the standards that are expected of us," says Jass, of the approximately 100 employees at FCHS. "Continuous improvement is

us with what, if anything, can be improved upon."

The surveyors do not determine whether or not FCHS receives its accreditation - that is done by the CCHSA council at a future date. They simply observe and submit a written report. A determination on accreditation usually takes approximately 45 days.

But Klein-Swormink says in her short visit she was impressed with the hospital and the way it functions.

"They have done a great deal of preparation in advance," she says. "They are taking this very seriously which is a very good sign. Also, the number of volunteers is incredible. That's a great thing to see."

"It is interesting to see what is happening in the various hospitals," says Cogswell. "Hospitals are all facing the same problems, such as funding, but they all still want to be at a certain level as far as their ability to serve their specific communities."

Four Counties Health Services Administrator Janak Jass, left, talks with Canadian Council on Health

Canadian Council on Health Services Accreditation
1730 St. Laurent Boulevard, Suite 430
Ottawa, ON Canada K1G 5L1

Conseil canadien d'agrément des services de santé
Tel.: (613) 738-3800 Fax: (613) 738-3755
www.cchsa.ca

Newspaper clipping of an accreditation review, but not a hospital discussed in the book.

To establish a relaxed atmosphere when interviewing larger groups, I often told them that I had wanted to bring the flavour of the Maritimes with me. It seemed impracticable to bring lobster, so instead I had with me the quintessential maritime snack: dulse. Then I would produce several packages, open one, take a large mouthful myself, and pass several packages around the room. Predictably, the tension would be broken, as many began to spit into their handkerchiefs. At times I was called the seaweed doctor.

First Nation's health care was a federal government responsibility and administered by Ottawa. I was privileged to survey several of these hospitals. Access roads to reserves, a provincial responsibility, were often poorly maintained, some not even paved. Roads inside the reserves, a federal responsibility, were much better. Many members of the hospital staffs were First Nations people who had left the area, obtained their training elsewhere, and returned to the community to run the hospital. The medical staff were an exception.

One excellent administrator told me her story. She had married a non-native, left the reservation at a young age, and had several children. They lived in British Columbia, and when her children began university, she did as well. She graduated from administration and planned to work near her new home. The Elders on her reserve, however, had another plan; they told her she had to return to the reserve and become the administrator of their hospital. She felt a duty to her people and went, knowing she would only see her west coast family on holidays. Once there, the Elders told her specifically what they wanted done in the hospital. At times she was obliged to reveal to them that the ideas they deemed necessary would not be allowed by the government in Ottawa. As a result, the native-born administrator was told by the Elders, "We thought you would say that—you are one of them now." On the flip side, there were occasions when the government officials in Ottawa informed the administrator of their expectations for the hospital, and she told them these were changes the Elders would not approve of. Their reply: "We knew you would say that—you are one of them."

Frequently, people across the country would tell me they did not believe the accreditation process was useful, accurate, or worth the cost. I knew hospitals that had considered discontinuing accreditation had been warned by their province that funding would be lost unless they could provide evidence that they were giving quality care. They were not compelled to use CCHSA, but equivalent proof of a hospital's competence was required. One provincial government decided to do their own reviews, but this policy soon developed political problems and was not continued. I remember an occasion when my survey team arrived at a small hospital and the administrator greeted us by announcing he did not believe in accreditation, but he would allow this one. Soon it became clear there was not one but two administrators—one for the hospital we were reviewing, and another, his superior, who had been given authority over this and two other local hospitals to develop cost-saving strategies. Previously, this senior administrator had made economies in the provincial grain industry by closing small-town elevators and centralizing grain management. Now it appeared he was there to find savings within the three hospitals.

While we were reviewing charts that evening, the nurse commented, "That is the third time you have said to me, 'I guess that is ok, but I would not have done it that way.'" She continued: "Why don't you go, yourself, and informally quiz the staff working at this hour of the night, and find out what is going on?" After I assured the evening staff that anything they told me would be off the record, and they would be anonymous, I learned there was a conflict within the medical staff. A team was coming the following week to do a review of this problem area which seemed to have possible political ramifications as well as a suspicion of malpractice. I also learned the staff had been threatened; anyone who informed the surveyors about the coming investigation would be fired.

I began the next morning session by stating the purpose of accreditation was to improve patient care and it was based on trust. I asked, "Why is this hospital hiding problems?"

The junior hospital administrator yelled at me, "Who told you? I'm gonna fire him! Who told you?"

The outburst stunned me. It was inappropriate then, and by present standards, completely unacceptable. The nurse surveyor intervened. "Nobody," she stated. "He found it in the charts."

She was correct. I had discovered their secret. At least one of the medical staff was being investigated the following week, apparently for incompetence.

The senior administrator, of grain elevator expertise, quieted his underling, and added, "We owe an apology and our thanks to this survey team . . . I think they have saved us a lot of problems."

At the time I was thinking how fortunate I was to work with such an excellent nurse, one of many I have met and worked with throughout my career. We recommended the hospital receive Accreditation, with a review of the medical staff in one year. The administrator realized surveyors could discover problems even when there was an active attempt to hide them by hospital administration. They continued their accreditation program.

Preceptor

Dalhousie University opened its Department of Family Medicine in 1968, and this new Department began its clinical programs in 1970. The Director, Dr. Don Brown, called me in May of 1972, twelve years after I had graduated, and asked me to become a preceptor for first, second-, and third-year medical students, Clinical Clerks (CC), as they were known. This family practice preceptor program had been so successful since its initiation in the city, it was being expanded into country. I would have four to six students a year, each for a two-week period, who would accompany me daily. CCs would spend two weeks with a city preceptor, as before, and an additional two weeks with a country preceptor, which would provide them with an overview of both urban and rural family medicine. It was the only period during their medical training where a student and a full-time instructor, the preceptor, worked one on one. I would be part of the initial group of rural preceptors. There was no financial remuneration, but I would become a part-time professor in the department of Family Medicine. To do my teaching I needed to allow more time with each patient, restricting the number of patients I could see each day. Given my years in practice, my membership in the College of Family Medicine since its inception, where I had been a provincial president, and my Certification by examination in the College, on September 10th,1972, I considered myself competent to contribute to the CCs' knowledge of family practice. I looked forward to meeting a group of future doctors, some of whom might be encouraged to return and practice here. I was pleased to accept.

Realizing that the CCs had already been taught specific illnesses and their treatments, I decided my role was to demonstrate how I dealt with patients, sorted their complaints, followed their response to treatment, and how to run an efficient practice. I used examples from my practice to answer their questions. My receptionist informed patients, when they made their appointments, that there would be a CC with me that week, so there would be no surprises. A few patients left my practice saying they refused to be used for teaching. Others were pleased I had been chosen to teach, and to be helpful, they asked for appointments during periods there was a CC. I overheard one woman while booking her routine pap smear, who informed the receptionist she did not mind having a student involved and, since other patients might not want a student, she thought she should help with teaching and requested her appointment at a time when a CC was present.

I demonstrated my methods of examining small children without frightening them. My office desk was not between me and my patients as many are, but on an angle to my chair to minimize any physical/emotional barrier. Patients sat on a padded custom built, medium size, high backed bench, which easily held a couple of adults and one or two small children. If a child required an abdominal examination, they could lie on the bench, their head secure on the parent's lap, rather than be deposited alone on a separate, frightening, pediatric examination table. Immunizations were given to children while they were held safe and secure by their mothers, usually caused little problem, especially when they knew they would be getting a balloon.

I warned each CC that they would be targets for salespeople who would encourage them to buy expensive homes, cars, cottages, trips— "You deserve it," they would be told. Then for years after beginning their practice, most of their earnings would be required to pay off these loans. I personally had been careful to avoid this type of debt, for which I was grateful when faced with the series of court cases about my daughter Suzanne's care.

I did, however, lose one patient early in my practice because of my efforts to avoid unnecessary purchases. I had arrived in my car, making a house call for a new patient. "You can't be much of a doctor to drive a vehicle like that," he remarked. "I'm going to change to a doctor who has a decent car." And he did.

As preceptors, we were instructed to find local accommodations for the CCs and told not to provide accommodations in our own homes. Each morning I collected the CC, and we spent the day together. At the end of the first day, one CC said he would prefer to drive me in his car and would pick me up the following morning. He appeared driving a new Corvette, which I admired, then went into my anti-debt rant. He replied he wanted the car now and would be able to afford to erase the debt in the future as he was going to become a cardiac surgeon; and now he is a cardiac surgeon.

Another CC told me he had not realized how easy it was to practice family medicine. I then realized I had not been demonstrating how an intimate knowledge of my patients' previous medical histories, memories of investigations and diagnostic tests, of illnesses treated and referrals made, contributed to good patient care. By changing my approach to teaching students, I was able to demonstrate how continuity of care is a valuable component of family medicine.

Another excellent CC confessed her first wish had been to become a veterinarian, but she was refused admission to veterinary college. She then decided to apply for medicine and was accepted. She now loved her medical studies.

The university organized annual preceptor meetings during which there were opportunities to mingle and learn from each other. At one meeting, a city preceptor introduced herself and asked my impression of a student we had shared. I immediately knew to whom she referred. He had concerned me, was difficult to manage, seemed immature, and lacked people skills. When left alone, he had children crying, adults resentful. I asked her about her time with him.

"I went home and cried each night," she confided.

His lack of interpersonal skills had been missed until we worked with him, one on one. We spoke to the director, who said the CC would be given extra help to improve his interpersonal skills.

Despite our short time together, I tried to have the CCs knowledgeable and comfortable interviewing patients, suturing simple wounds, doing intubations, setting up intravenous lines, monitoring anaesthetics. The surgeon allowed them to be part of some surgical procedures.

I learned a great deal from my students, as I was reminded a few months ago when I received a call from an out-of-province physician who was visiting Halifax. I started to explain I was retired, no longer in practice, and would not be able to help him. He interrupted to say he was calling to thank me for saving his wife's life. He went on to remind me I had delivered her, and because of neonatal jaundice had immediately transferred her to the children's hospital for phototherapy. This was a new therapy one of my CCs had discussed with me, prior to it becoming general knowledge. The doctors at the children's hospital had informed the family my rapid referral saved her life. How kind of her physician husband to call me to bring me up to date.

Toast to the 2010 Dalhousie Medical School Graduation Class15

The following is a modified version of the speech I gave, and it contains some medical terms that were relevant to them, and to me.

As the representative of the class of 1960, I am pleased to be asked to give the toast to the graduating class. When Vonda called, I asked what the traditional topic had been. "Changes in medicine during the past fifty years," she replied. I asked how long I had for this huge task. "Five minutes," she answered. I will do my best.

Our Graduation Class consisted of fifty students, but your class now has 105, three times as many. We had forty-six men and four women, while you have fifty-four men and fifty-one women, which gives a much better balance. You are free to do your internship anywhere, but we did not have that choice. During our internship, we were paid seventy-five dollars a month and murmurs of "slave labour" could be heard from members of my class. My father, who graduated in 1932, believed this was a reasonable amount because he had received seventy-five dollars for an entire year of internship. Speaking of income, the fee schedule in place when I began practice in 1963 suggested three dollars for an office visit. In Aylesford we charged $2.50 because it was a less affluent area compared to Halifax. When I began, the fee schedule paid physicians by the procedure, not by the qualifications of the physician. For example, the fee for a hernia repair was the same for general practitioners as it was for surgeons.

Our medical school experience was very different from yours. It began with mandatory re-vaccination for smallpox, and one for tuberculosis. We were given detailed lectures on how to do an appendectomy and make emergency burr holes for subdural haematoma to relieve pressure on the brain. An important part of my paediatric internship rotation was instruction on tonsillectomies and adenoidectomies (T&A procedures). These were the type of emergency and routine procedures we might be required to do. We were also, at times, used as "volunteers." At one of our physiology classes, conducted by an anaesthesiologist and several residents, we were asked to volunteer for a gas anaesthesia induction to experience what our future patients would experience. Was this a learning experience for us or a teaching experience for the residents?

Attendance for one particular lecture was optional. A brave gynecologist furtively gave us a brief, off-the-record lecture on contraception. He was not on the university staff and because there was no introduction, we did not even know his name. We were informed that no notes were to be taken and there would be no examination questions from this lecture. In fact, this gynecologist was breaking the law. Contraception was not formally legalized in Canada until 1969. It was illegal to give contraceptive advice at the time of the lecture and for the first few years when I was in practice. The birth control pill was on the market, but only as a drug to control menstrual periods.

We were given a Vademecum when we graduated, a book that listed and described the several hundred drugs then approved for use in Canada. Over the last fifty years, what is now known as the Compendium of Pharmaceuticals and Specialties (or CPS) has increased in size to more than 2,700 pages. This number does not, of course, include the homeopathic and herbal medications now available in most drugstores.

I will paraphrase Sir William Osler, who wrote the medical text-book my grandfather used, who once said something to the effect that a young physician begins their work life with twenty drugs for each disease, and the older one ends their career with one drug for twenty diseases. He also believed that one of the first duties of the physician was to educate the masses not to take medicines (1902). Judging from the size of the CPS and Osler's textbook, our generation has not done very well at minimizing drug usage. It is now your turn. Perhaps you can do better.

A local physician, Dr. Kinsman, and I had arranged the first "sign out" system in the valley to allow each of us more free time. To provide good care, we discussed cases we would both be seeing. This did not, however, impress some of the local population as indicated by the following story. One evening, Dr. Kinsman told me that, because of being overtired, he had inadvertently criticized a mother for not calling him earlier to see her sick child. She had hung up on him and he believed soon she would call me. He wanted to be certain I would go to see the child, whom he knew to be sick. Sure enough, the phone rang almost immediately and off I went. As I entered the house, the child's mother said to a neighbour, who was there commiserating with her, "It's like I said: Dr. Kinsman is the best doctor, but if you have Dr. Cogswell at least you die happy."

We all know the world of medicine today, so I will describe the world of medicine when I began. As I did part-time anaesthesia, I will use it as my example. I gave my first anaesthetic for my father when I was about fifteen years old. I frequently asked to go on his "calls," but this time he asked me to go with him. When we entered the house, a woman was on the kitchen floor with her arm in an awkward position. Dad examined her and determined she had dislocated her shoulder. He said, "David will put you to sleep, and I will set it." Dad had his obstetrical bag with him and produced an anaesthetic mask and chloroform. He then instructed me in the procedure. As soon as she was asleep, he reduced the shoulder and put the arm in a sling. We monitored her and left when she had fully recovered. On the way home I asked why he had not taken her to the hospital, X-rayed the shoulder, had another doctor give the anaesthetic, and set the shoulder more conveniently. He explained that the family had little money and could not afford the cost of hospitalization and another doctor's bill. It would have ruined their Christmas.

When I began practice in the valley, neither the equipment nor the skill to use it were available to perform intubations. Chloroform was the standard induction method and ether was the standard maintenance anaesthetic for T&A procedures. Every operating room had a T&A machine which was essentially an air pump. The air blew through a jar of ether, the vaporized ether through a catheter hooked to the side of the patient's mouth, which was inhaled by the patient. Another jar on the air intake side of the pump collected secretions suctioned from the tonsillar bed by the anaesethologist. Surgery was considered more important than the particulars of the required anaesthetic, so anaesthetists were expected to make themselves useful by also assisting the surgeon.

This is a window into the state of the kind of medical practice I entered fifty years ago. Some day one of you will be asked to give a toast to the class of 2060. Then you may be asked to give a summary of changes in medicine during your fifty years in practice. Just think . . . together you and I will have participated in the changes in medicine for over one hundred years—amazing!

I trust you will enjoy the practice of medicine during your fifty years as much as I have during mine.

Cogswell Geneology

John   COGSWELL   Born   1592.................   Elizabeth
THOMPSON. Born circa 1594
Westbury Leigh Wiltshire, England   Westbury Leigh
   Wiltshire, England
Died 29/Nov/1669 Ipswich Mass Died 2/Jun/1676 Ipswich Mass
John COGSWELL...Born25/Jul/1622......." Miss
   ROGERS" Born.......
Westbury Leigh Wiltshire, England
Died 27/Sept/1653 at sea........................ Died 1652
Samuel COGSWELL.............................Suzanna HAVEN
Born 1651   Born 24/Apr/1653 Saybrook Conn
Died 'Prior to 1701'   Died -------
Samuel COGSWELL----------------------------Anne DENISON
Born 3/Aug/1677 Saybrook Conn   Born 1655/1669
   Stonington Conn
Died 21/Mar/1753 Lebanon Conn   Died 17/Jun/1753
   Lebanon Conn
Hezekiah COGSWELL........................... Suzanna BAILEY
Born 19/Feb/1709 Saybrook Conn   Born 1711
   Mansfield Conn
Died circa1806 Cornwallis, N.S. Died 1801 Annapolis, N.S.
Oliver COGSWELL...............................Abigail ELLS
Born 1740 Lebanon Conn   Born   (unknown)

Died 14/May/1783 Cornwallis, N.S.　　Died circa 1840

They lived 'Cogswell homestead' Canard street

Samuel COGSWELL...........................Emma LOVELESS

Born 29/Dec/1774 Cornwallis N.S.　　Born 2/Jan/1786
　　Greenwich, N.S.

Died 6/Jun/1841 Horton, N.S.　Died 29/Dec/1873 Horton, N.S.

Oliver Hezekiah COGSWELL .... Rebecca CROWE

Born 21/Feb/1806 Horton N.S.　Born 16/Oct/1809

Died　　Died

They lived in Morristown, N.S.

Abner W...COGSWELL....................... Louisa
　　A. TURNER

Born 28/Dec/1833 Morristown　Born　　Feb/1835

Died 16/Mar/1921 Morristown　Died 23/Sept/1921 Morristown

They resided in Cornwallis, N.S.

Eidson Whitter COGSWELL.........................Naomi
　　Elizabeth NICHOLS

Born 2/SEP/1875 Morristown, N.S.....................Born 5/
　　April/1881 Nicholsville, N.S.

Died 5/May/1948 Berwick, N.S. ....Died 10/
　　June/1927 Morristown, N S

Laverne Eidson COGSWELL.........................Kathleen
　　Eleanor KILLAM

Born 23/May/1907 Morristown, N.S.................... Born 30/
　　Dec/1910 Kinsman Corners, N.S.

David Laverne COGSWELL.........................Heide
　　Anna WENKHAUSEN

Born 20/Oct/1936 Berwick, N.S.Born 15/April/1938
　　Berlin Germany

Died　　Died 16/July/2014 Kentville, N.S.

Endnotes

1. Kathleen Eleanor Cogswell, 'Western Kings Memorial Hospital, 1922-1982.' R S. Babcock Ltd, New Minas, NS; 64 pp. See also: '1907, The Last Smallpox Epidemic,' *Berwick Register* Sept. 26, 1990, p.11: and 'Dr. Harold E. Killam-A Country Physician.' *Nova Scotia Medical Journal* 1992, Vol. 71/3, p. 147.

2. Medical Service Insurance (MSI) began in Nova Scotia April1,1969.

3. Kathleen, my mother, earned her bachelor's degree in history from Dalhousie University in 1930, and a master's degree in History (*sum com laude*) in 1931 from University of Toronto. Her thesis topic was the life of Lord Dalhousie.

4. Pat J. Hampsey, 'Berwick Camp Meeting Grounds'; see p. 16 in: *Exit 15: A History of Berwick*; publications date and printer unknown.

5. The Valley Branch of the Nova Scotia Medical Society met four times a year at various locations between Digby and Windsor.

6. Dr. Paul Kinsman was a family doctor who practised in various locations, including Aylesford and Wolfville.

7. Grandfather Killam's medical kit (circa 1914) is in my possession.

8. Thomas Chandler Haliburton, wrote a weekly newspaper series with the character *Sam Slick*, an American Clock salesman, as a

cautionary tale to the local populace about the slippery American salesman. This was years after the arrival of the Nichols.

9. *Canadian Art: The Thomson Collection at the Art Gallery of Ontario* (Paul Holberton Publishing, Nov. 1 2008), p-c-715, "LT. Alfred Torrensand His Wife in Front of The Citadel, c. 1854" by Cornelius Krieghoff.

10. Carol Harris, author of many journal articles, holds a PhD in Education from the University of Victoria, and she is also a long-time dog enthusiast.

11. Wolfville textile specialist Karen Diadick Casselman is of the opinion that the dyes used to colour the handwoven woollen edging around the wolf rug are derived from natural sources, and that the weaving itself appears to be in a style reminiscent of "circa 1850." '(Pers. Comm, 2020.) Her books include *Craft of the Dyer* (University of Toronto Press, 1980).

12. Halifax historian Sharon MacDonald's books include *Old Nova Scotia Quilts* (Nova Scotia Museum 1995); Ms. MacDonald's expertise also extends to hooked mats. Sharon is of the view that the weaving on the woolen edging dates to mid-nineteenth century, and she confirms the dyes appear not to be derived from commercial products. (Pers. Comm, 2018.)

13. Ruth Holmes Whitehead is acknowledged authority on native culture; author of more than twenty books, her interpretation of the carriage rug was particularly useful; firstly, as she had "not seen anything like it" in her research of numerous collections within Canada and beyond. Secondly, she believed the piece to be "a trade item," likely from the west, or northern regions, where wolf pelts would have been available to create "items of great prestige." (Pers. Comm, 2018).

14. *Canadian Art: The Thomson Collection at the Art Gallery of Ontario* (Paul Holberton Publishing, Nov. 1 2008), p-c-304, "Breaking Up of a Country Ball in Canada, c. 1857" by Cornelius Krieghoff.

15. This portion of the book is based on my "Toast to the graduating medical class of 2010" which was published in *VoxMeDal* (Dalhousie Medical Alumni Magazine), Summer/Fall 2010, p. 18 David Cogswell, MD CCFP FCFP.

Bibliography

Gorenflo, L.G.,1942. "Building the Biloxi Dinghy." *The Young Craftsman.* a book first published by Popular Mechanics, Chicago, and later imprinted by General Publishing Co. Limited, Toronto, in 1942.

Kitz, Janet. 2008. *Shattered City: the Halifax Explosion:* Nimbus p. 63.

Osler, William. 1902. *Principles and Practise of Medicine: Textbook of Medicine.* Fifth edition. Appleton, New York

Letters written to Laverne, my father, by his mother my grandmother, Naomi Cogswell (Nichols) are in the possession of my sister, Mary Graham, Berwick.

Hampsey, Pat J. 'Berwick Camp Meeting Grounds'; see p. 16 in: *Exit 15: A History of Berwick*; publications date and printer unknown.

Vogel, Lauren. *Culture of Bullying in Medicine Starts at the Top,* Canadian Medical Journal, CMAJ 2018 December 10;190:E1459-60. doi: 10.1503/cmaj.109-5690

Johnson, Barb. *Could You be a Bully?,* doctors NS 2019, Vol. 18/7, p. 12.

McKenzie-Sutter, Holly. *Bullying, gender bias, harassment tolerated: report,* The Chronicle Herald, July 18, 2018.

Middlemiss, Nicola. *Doctor wins landmark workplace bullying lawsuit,* https://www.hcamag.com/ca/news/general/doctor-wins-landmark-workplace-bullying-lawsuit/127937, June 24, 2016.

Creery, E.A., Lieutenant Commander R.C.N., *The Autocar May 13/1949 p.450.* "Rolls-Royce Leave Three Canadian Naval Officers Go Home and Back (8000) Miles in a 1919 Silver Ghost."

CPSIA information can be obtained
at www.ICGtesting.com
Printed in the USA
LVHW101945281022
731818LV00020B/816/J

9 781039 144538